Healing From Sexual Trauma

Shawn E. Ellis

TABLE OF CONTENTS

WEATHERING THE STORM: THE JOURNEY OF HEALING FROM SEXUAL TRAUMA 1

CHAPTER 1: CONCEPTUAL FRAMEWORK 2

    SEXUAL VIOLENCE AMONG UNDERREPRESENTED GROUPS 2

    SEXUAL TRAUMA 6

    IMPACTS OF SEXUAL VIOLENCE 8

    SEXUAL TRAUMA AND CULTURAL CONSIDERATIONS 11

        Cultural Betrayal Trauma Theory *12*

    PROCESSING SEXUAL TRAUMA 14

        Relationship to Perpetrator *16*

        Resiliency Skills *17*

        Advocacy *19*

        Social Connection *20*

        Justice *21*

        Forgiveness *21*

        Socioeconomic and Cultural Background *25*

    SUMMARY OF THE CONCEPTUAL FRAMEWORK 25

    STATEMENT OF THE PROBLEM 26

CHAPTER 2: METHODOLOGY 29

    INTERPRETIVE FRAMEWORK 30

        Critical qualitative inquiry *31*

        Social constructivism *32*

       Charmaz's constructivist grounded theory.. 33

       Grounded theory and situational analysis 35

ONTOLOGY.. 36

EPISTEMOLOGY 37

AXIOLOGY... 39

METHODOLOGY 41

    Research Question 42

    Sampling and Participant Selection Procedures 42

    Data Gathering Method 48

    Data Analysis Procedures... 52

    Procedures for Establishing Trustworthiness 54

       Inquiry Audit.. 55

       Institutional Review Board (IRB). 55

       Prolonged Engagement 56

       Member check... 57

       Triangulation. 58

       Memo 58

       Journaling.. 59

    Researcher positionality and reflexivity.. 59

SUMMARY OF THE METHODOLOGY.. 61

CHAPTER 3: FIRST-ROUND ANALYSIS 62

DESCRIPTION OF PARTICIPANTS... 64

EMERGING PARTICIPANT EXPERIENCES 66

Sociocultural contexts 67

    Family culture and socialization 68

    Encounters with the system... 76

    Emotional burden 82

Identity exploration and formation 86

    Gender identity.. 87

    Sexual orientation.. 90

    Racial identity 92

    Disability identity.. 94

Pre-trauma self and relationships.. 96

    Sense of Self.. 96

    Relationship with the perpetrator 98

    Relationship with trusted others.. 98

Responding to trauma 99

    Somatic responses 101

    Emotional responses.. 103

    Psychological responses.. 110

    Behavioral responses... 127

The Perpetrator... 133

    The perpetrator's identity 133

    Perpetrator's attempt to contact the survivor 135

Disclosure 137

    Intrapersonal considerations of disclosure 138

    Interpersonal outcomes of disclosure 141

    Moments of relief and empowerment *147*

ROUND ONE EMERGING PROCESSES 151

    Authenticity leads to positive trauma response and moments of relief 152

    Acceptance by others facilitates identity exploration and formation 153

    Encounters with the system shapes decisions of reporting sexual violence 154

    Processes within responding to trauma 154

SUMMARY OF FIRST-ROUND INTERVIEW 156

CHAPTER 4: SECOND-ROUND ANALYSES 161

REVIEW OF PROCEDURES 161

DATA ANALYSES 163

EXPERIENCES OF SEXUAL TRAUMA 164

    Sociocultural contexts and socialization *168*

        Family culture and upbringings. 169

        Identity socializations. 170

        Identity exploration and formation. 172

        Pre-trauma self and relationships 177

    Power and privilege *180*

        Aggressor's power and privilege. 181

        Survivor's power and privilege 191

        Emotional burden 196

    Trauma response *200*

    Disclosure *210*

Moments of relief 213

    Internal relief. 215

    External relief 217

EMERGING PROCESSES 221

    Process of internalizing blame to externalizing blame 224

    Exposure to new and inclusive cultures 226

    Process of the shift in understanding of consent 229

    Recognition of sexual encounter as violence 232

    Time with intentional effort 233

    Triggers lead to negative somatic and emotional responses of trauma 236

    Safety within the sociocultural contexts leads to moments of relief 239

    Sociocultural contexts and socialization shape the power and privilege 241

    Positive disclosure outcomes lead to moments of relief and positive trauma response 243

CONCLUSIONS OF SECOND ROUND ANALYSIS 245

CHAPTER 5: WEATHERING THE STORM: THE JOURNEY OF HEALING FROM SEXUAL TRAUMA 247

    THE BOAT 248

    SHIFT IN UNDERSTANDING OF CONSENT 252

    RECOGNIZING SEXUAL ENCOUNTER AS VIOLENCE 253

    TIME AND INTENTIONAL EFFORT 254

    EXPOSURE TO NEW AND INCLUSIVE CULTURES 254

    TRAUMA RESPONSE 255

    DISCLOSURE 265

- Moments of relief 266
- Summary 267

CHAPTER 6: TRUSTWORTHINESS, LIMITATIONS, AND IMPLICATIONS 269

- Establishing Trustworthiness 273
  - *Member checking* 273
    - Member checking results 274
  - *Triangulation* 276
  - *Peer debriefing* 277
  - *Inquiry auditing* 278
  - *Generating thick and rich descriptions* 278
  - *Reflexivity* 279
- Achieving saturation 281
- Implications 283
  - *For survivors of sexual trauma* 283
  - *For mental health service providers* 285
  - *For educators and supervisors of mental health professionals* 286
  - *For members of the justice system* 287
  - *For friends, family and/or others in relationship with survivors* 288
- Future research 288
- Conclusion 289

WEATHERING THE STORM: THE JOURNEY OF HEALING FROM SEXUAL TRAUMA

Nearly 1 in 4 women and 1 in 26 men in the United States (Basile et al., 2022) and 6% of women across the globe (15 years and older) have experienced sexual violence in their lifetime (WHO, 2021). Studies (e.g., CDC, n.d.; HRC, 2019; RAINN, 2020) showed that higher rates of sexual violence are reported among individuals identifying as members of an underrepresented group. Scientific studies conducted on the impact of sexual violence and trauma show the mental and physical health issues experienced by survivors following this encounter (e.g., van der Kolk, 2014). Identifying a comprehensive framework of the experience and process of healing from sexual trauma as it applies to survivors within underrepresented groups is essential to helping address and heal these mental and physical health issues.

CHAPTER 1: CONCEPTUAL FRAMEWORK

This chapter provides an overview of the prevalence of sexual violence among individuals identifying as members of underrepresented groups based on their racial, gender, sexual orientation, and disability identities. Common definitions of terms of sexual violence are clarified and the impact of sexual violence on survivors' wellbeing and cultural considerations are discussed. I will end this chapter by discussing strategies that help survivors process their experience with sexual trauma and the gaps in the literature that were intended to be answered by this dissertation study.

Sexual Violence among Underrepresented Groups

The United States' Centers for Disease Control and Prevention (CDC; n.d.) reported that sexual violence is a public health problem that leads to both physical and psychological injuries. On an individual level, some of the possible consequences of sexual violence are posttraumatic stress disorder and reproductive, gastrointestinal, cardiovascular, and sexual health issues (CDC, n.d.). In addition, some survivors of sexual violence experience lower cortisol levels and attention deficits as compared to a control group (Quidé et al., 2018). On a societal level, the public health interventions required to address the needs of survivors are expensive and include medical costs, costs involving criminal justice activities and lost productivity due to job loss, reduced performance or being unable to work (CDC; n.d.).

In the United States, nearly 1 in 4 women and 1 in 26 men have experienced a completed or attempted rape in their lifetime (Basile et al., 2022). At the college level, research indicates that 1 in 5 women report being a victim of sexual violence (Muehlenhar et al., 2017). The Association of American Universities' (AAU) report on Campus Climate Survey on Sexual Assault and Misconduct revealed that the rate of nonconsensual sexual contact by physical force and/or inability to consent was higher for both women and non-women identifying individuals in gender underrepresented groups (Cantor, 2020). In addition, Tjaden & Thoennes (2000) reported that ten percent of surveyed women had experienced sexual violence after the age of 18 (Tjaden & Thoennes, 2000) and the World Health Organization (WHO, 2021) reported that 6% of women across the globe (15 years and older) have experienced sexual violence by a non-partner at least once in their lifetime. The latter report indicated that the number would even be higher if sexual violence within an intimate relationship was considered (WHO, 2021).

Although most reports focus on women survivors of sexual violence, individuals identifying across the gender spectrum, and those belonging to other underrepresented group are subjected to sexual violence every year and may be at greater risk of becoming victims of sexual violence (e.g., CDC, n.d.; Human Rights Campaign [HRC], 2019; Rape, Abuse & Incest National Network [RAINN], 2020). For instance, the CDC states that both men and women with disabilities are at greater risk of sexual violence compared to those without a disability (CDC, n.d.). Among gender and sexual underrepresented groups, the Rape, Abuse, and Incest National Network (RAINN, 2020) indicated that transgender, genderqueer and/or nonconforming students are at a higher risk of becoming sexually victimized. For instance, HRC (2019) indicated 27% of transgender and gender expansive youth and 14% of cisgender queer youth were found to have been subjected to sexual violence. Similarly, Martin-Storey, et al. (2018) found that college students in Canada who identify with sexual and gender minorities reported significantly higher sexual violence encounters compared to students who identify with dominant identities.

Studies indicate that racially underrepresented groups are disproportionally impacted by sexual violence and its consequences. For example, Native Americans are at greater risk of sexual violence compared to non-Native men and women (RAINN, 2020). According to The National Intimate Partner and Sexual Violence Survey (NISVS), 49.5% of American Indian/Alaska Native women experienced some form of sexual violence (Smith et al., 2017). Specifically, Rosay (2016) indicated that 56.1% of American Indian/Alaska Native women and 27.5% of American Indian/Alaska Native men reported a sexually violent experience at some point in their lives. Moreover, 35.5% of non-Hispanic Black women, 26.9% of Hispanic women, and 22.9% of Asian/ Pacific Islander women experienced some form of sexual violence in their lifetime (Rosay, 2016). These prevalence rates indicate the need for more studies and interventions designed to address the needs of survivors of sexual violence not only in underrepresented race-based groups but also in survivors from underrepresented gender, sexual orientation, and disability groups.

Despite the significantly higher number of reports of sexual violence among underrepresented groups, the CDC (n.d.) indicated that many sexual violence cases are not reported due to feeling threatened with additional harm or because survivors do not think they will be able to receive help. This hesitation to report sexual violence is amplified in racial underrepresented communities (RAINN, 2020; Wiesboeck, 2020). For example, Wiesboeck (2020) found that Arkansas counties that have the largest percentage of underrepresented residents (Black, Hispanic, and non-U.S. born) were the least likely to report sexual offenses. The study stipulates that the lack of reporting can be associated with the limited access to services and/or prejudiced treatments of underrepresented groups after reporting sex offenses (Wiesboeck, 2020). In line with this explanation, RAINN (2020) reported that, despite experiencing higher rates of sexual violence as compared with their White counterparts, Black women are less likely to report their experience to the justice system due to the negative experiences they personally have, or their family/community has had with law enforcement. It is important that research studies and intervention strategies consider the role of intercultural and intracultural relationships in reporting and processing the experience of sexual violence.

One theory that highlights the role of culture as a key factor to understanding trauma in underrepresented groups is The Cultural Betrayal Trauma Theory (CBTT) developed by Jennifer Gomez in 2012. The CBTT portrays the shared understanding and camaraderie that people in underrepresented groups develop as a protection against societal oppression and trauma. This intracultural trust and loyalty play a part in how individuals process and disclose interpersonal trauma, especially when the perpetrator is supposed to share the intracultural solidarity to which they subscribe (Gomez, 2018). According to Gomez (2019), close to 50% of women reported that their ethnicity has made it difficult to disclose the violence they experienced. This leads survivors to minimize, dissociate, and/ or deny the trauma. Underrepresented group members may feel a sense of responsibility to protect their entire community and in turn, this cultural pressure contributes to the mental health problems experienced by survivors of trauma (Gomez, 2019). As a result, efforts to address the mental health needs of survivors of sexual trauma need to integrate the cultural and systemic factors that add to the challenges faced by survivors.

Understanding the process of surviving, and the journey of navigating the mental and physical health issues for underrepresented survivors of sexual violence, would contribute significantly to the services provided to these survivors. The purpose of this grounded theory dissertation was to explore the journey of sexual trauma survivors who identify as gender, sexual, ability, and race minorities.

Sexual Trauma

A variety of terms are used to describe the use of force in an attempt or act of unwanted sexual advances by perpetrators. Recognizing the importance of services, guidelines, advocacy, and policies related to addressing sexual violence, different organizations have created their own definitions to address the issue.

The WHO (2012) broadly defines sexual violence as *"any sexual act, attempt to obtain a sexual act, unwanted sexual comments or advances, or acts to traffic or otherwise directed against a person's sexuality using coercion, by any person regardless of their relationship to the victim, in any setting, including but not limited to home and work"* (p. 2). RAINN (2020) refers to the term sexual violence as an *"all encompassing, non-legal term that refers to crimes like sexual assault, rape and sexual abuse."* Other organizations use the word *sexual assault* instead of *sexual violence* and highlight the importance of consent by the victim at the time of the attempt or an act involving sexual advances. For instance, the Department of Justice (DoJ, 2021) describes sexual assault as *"any nonconsensual sexual act proscribed by Federal, tribal, or State law, including when the victim lacks capacity to consent."* In addition, the CDC states sexual violence as *"any sexual act that is committed or attempted by a perpetrator without the consent of an individual"* (Basile et al., 2014, p. 11). Behaviorally, the words *sexual violence* can encompass different types of actions or attempts including rape, being forced to penetrate someone else, sexual coercion, and unwanted sexual contact (Smith et al., 2018).

As shown in the above definitions, sexual violence is a broad term that incorporates varied experiences of victims. The NSVRC (2021) states that, at the beginning of each study, researchers need to identify the specific terminology to be used in the study and the behaviors included in that specific investigation. Proper attunement to the terminologies used in a study are relevant especially when determining the prevalence of survivors of unwanted sexual advances. For this study, this operational definition of sexual violence is proposed:

> *Sexual violence is an act and/or an attempt of unwanted sexual advances involving force or coercion which occurs without the consent of the survivor. Sexual violence can happen in any setting, and the perpetrator(s) may nor may not have a preexisting relationship with the victim.*

Moreover, individuals who have reported experiences of sexual violence will be addressed throughout this study as "survivors/survivors of sexual violence" to help connect the personal path of the survival journey.

Sexual violence has multifaced consequences on the physical and mental health of the survivors (Campbell et al., 2009; Durà-Vilà et al., 2013; Ha et al., 2019; Quidé et al., 2018; Saint & Sinko, 2019; van der Kolk, 2014). These psychological and physical consequences are reported to be significantly higher in individuals who identify with underrepresented groups compared to those in non-underrepresented groups (Paquette et al., 2021). Paquette et al (2021) reported that gender non-binary/transgender and sexual underrepresented undergraduate university students experienced the highest levels of sexual violence and trauma symptoms (e.g., hypervigilance, flashbacks, avoidance, or dissociation) as a result of the sexual violence compared with their counterparts who identify as cisgender women and men.

The survival journey from sexual trauma is often characterized by a pendulum swinging between successful intervention strategies helpful to the survivor (e.g., Campbell et al., 2009; Saint & Sinko, 2019), and the ongoing emotional, cognitive, and behavioral challenges in the aftermath of experiencing sexual violence (e.g., Freedman & Enright, 2017; Prieto-Ursúa, 2021; Worthington, 2005). To fully understand this journey of deep emotional experiences, it is valuable to learn the meaning the survivors place on the journey – encompassing the helpful and challenging aspects of the journey. A framework/theory of the experience will be a valuable resource for tailoring survivor support. To this end, grounded theory was used to guide this study through identifying the social contexts that shape researcher positionality and critical stance, and participants co-constructed knowledge on the meaning and process of surviving sexual violence.

Creswell and Poth (2018) stated that qualitative research creates an opportunity for researchers to implement an interpretative naturalistic approach. The authors also illustrated that qualitative research helps make the experiences of individuals visible and creates an opportunity to transform world views. This implies that in qualitative research, the researcher studies the world in its natural settings, and attempts to make sense of and interpret the experiences based on the meaning people bring to them (Creswell & Poth, 2018). For survivors of sexual violence, understanding the impact that the violating experience has on them and how they choose to address the impact will guide physical and mental health services that are designed to help those in need.

Impacts of Sexual Violence

Survivors of sexual violence often experience significant mental and physical health issues as part of the survival process (van der Kolk, 2014). Prieto-Ursúa (2021) indicated that experiences of sexual violence can be traumatizing and stigmatizing, often leading victims to feelings of hopelessness. Life after an experience of sexual violence is often associated with compromised emotional, physical, and relational health and wellbeing (Freedman & Enright, 2017; Prieto-Ursúa, 2021; Worthington, 2005). Multiple studies reported that the trauma response of survivors of sexual violence may include shame, anger, and self-blame (Campbell et al., 2009; Durà-Vilà et al., 2013; Ha, Bae, & Hyun, 2019; Saint & Sinko, 2019). Somatic symptoms were also reported as one of the most prevalent mental health problems experienced by survivors of sexual violence (Hemma et al., 2018). Quidé et al (2018) reported that lower levels of cortisol, attentional deficits and functional brain modification when processing emotional materials were observed in women who survived sexual violence compared to those who have not experienced sexual violence. The consistent exposure to anger and fear due to the traumatic experience can also lead to muscle tension and spasm, back pain, headaches, and fibromyalgia (van der Kolk, 2014). Clinically, studies reported that the consequences of sexual violence may include some or all symptoms of general trauma: posttraumatic stress disorder, depression, anxiety, fear, substance abuse disorders, and suicidal ideation (Campbell et al., 2009; Hemma et al., 2018; Saint & Sinko, 2019). In 2007, Wuest et al.'s study among 309 adult English-speaking female participants revealed that child abuse history and sexual assault history were associated with higher levels of use of pain medications, antidepressants, and psychotropic medications. This finding reiterates the negative impact of sexual violence on the survivor's mental and physical health.

Impacts of sexual violence on mental health are wide-ranging and include shock, distress, anger, mistrust, withdrawal, and lower self-esteem. For example, Durà-Vilà et al. (2013), in a study among nuns who experienced sexual violence, found that the post-violence reactions included shock, distress, and anger. Participants also reported mistrust and withdrawal. Self-doubt — mainly doubting the innocence of self—was also identified as one of the struggles of the nuns (Durà-Vilà et al., 2013). Campbell et al. (2009) found that self-blame was one of the major post-assault experiences for survivors. In this review study, African American and Hispanic sexual assault survivors reported higher levels of self-blame than their White counterparts. The review also indicated that African American women were more likely to feel they were at risk of being victimized and sexually assaulted than their White counterparts. The feeling of not being valued due to preexisting race-based biases lead to internalizing a cultural blame that was then associated with lower self-esteem levels (Cambell et al, 2009).

Intracultural community dynamics also influence rates of reporting and accessing support by sexual trauma survivors in underrepresented group. For example, Gomez and Gobin (2019) reported that Black women's and girls' experience of oppression and racial trauma complicated their decision to report Black male perpetrators. The survivors faced the dilemma of either reporting one of their community members to a system that had historically mistreated them or refrain from disclosures and dealing with the mental health issues associated with the aftermath of the sexual violence, thereby protecting the trust within the intracultural community (Gomez & Gobin, 2019). The same study indicated that interracial sexual trauma is harmful to Black women and girls. However, sexual trauma as a cultural betrayal trauma is reported to be the predictor of more negative psychological consequences (Gomez & Gobin, 2019).

Based on a survey conducted among ethnic underrepresented undergraduate students, Gomez (2016) revealed that 43% of the participants reported within group victimization contributing to trauma outcomes such as PTSD, psychotic symptoms, and hypervigilance. This is indicative of the intersectionality of socioeconomic and cultural factors adding to the complexities of the negative effects of sexual violence.

Sexual Trauma and Cultural Considerations

The impacts of sexual violence, specifically as experienced by individuals who identify with underrepresented groups, revealed the importance of integrating the intersection of identities when examining the process of surviving sexual trauma. The social position of individuals that place them in an underrepresented status could contribute to the heightened stress they experience (Meyer, 2003). The stigma and prejudice individuals experience because of their position in the social structure impact how they process their experiences with trauma (Meyer, 2003).

In 2014, youth surveillance information on physical dating violence victimization revealed that sexually underrepresented youth experience significantly higher levels of physical dating violence compared to their heterosexual counterparts (Luo et al., 2014). Similarly, Sigurvinsdottir and Ullman (2016) indicated that bisexual women who were sexually assaulted reported greater symptoms of depression and posttraumatic stress disorder (PTSD) compared to heterosexual women, and in this study, symptoms of depression started similarly for all ethnic groups. However, Black women experienced a faster decline across the duration of the study. In this study, based on three yearly survey responses of sexual victimizations and trauma responses, Black bisexual women reported the highest PTSD symptoms as compared to non-Black bisexual women (Sigurvinsdottir & Ullman, 2016).

In another study, Whitton et al. (2021) reported that Black and Latinx participants experienced significantly higher rates of intimate partner violence (IPV) as compared to

White women participants. In this study, structural inequality variables, economic stress, and ethnic/racial discrimination were found to be associated with an increased exposure to intimate partner violence. As a result, future studies focusing on the role of stress due to being a member of underrepresented group in processing sexual violence for underrepresented trauma survivors would be valuable (Sigurvinsdottir & Ullman, 2016).

Cultural Betrayal Trauma Theory

Cultural Betrayal Trauma Theory (CBTT) was first coined by Jennifer M. Gomez, who theorized that individuals who experienced trauma are also impacted by social cultural contexts (Gomez, 2019). Societal discrimination and oppression towards underrepresented groups provide a context to understand how individuals with traumatic experiences process and heal from the trauma. Gomez (2019) revealed that the intra-culture that values honesty and protection of its members guide those individuals' decisions on whether or not to disclose abuse. The intracultural trust, defined as a "connection, attachment, and dependence, similar to racial loyalty" (Gomez, 2019, p. 2) is developed by minorities to "protect themselves and each other from discrimination and other societal trauma" (p. 2). Gomez (2019) further clarifies that the existence of this loyalty and solidarity within a minority culture creates an intercultural pressure leading victims not to disclose mental health issues related to victimization and not to cooperate with the legal system. CBTT hypothesizes that for cultural betrayal to occur the perpetrator is likely to be within the same underrepresented group. CBTT stipulates that the cultural context can result in outcomes such as internalized prejudice, cultural pressure, and changes to ethnic identity. In response to this, Gomez (2018) adapted the ecological systems model for CBTT to indicate how an individual in an underrepresented group might experience sexual trauma as more complex and multifaceted than their majority counterpart(s). Please see Figure 1 for a visual depiction of Bronfenbrenner's Ecological Systems Model adapted for CBTT.

Figure 1

Bronfenbrenner's Ecological Systems Model Adapted for Cultural Betrayal Trauma Theory

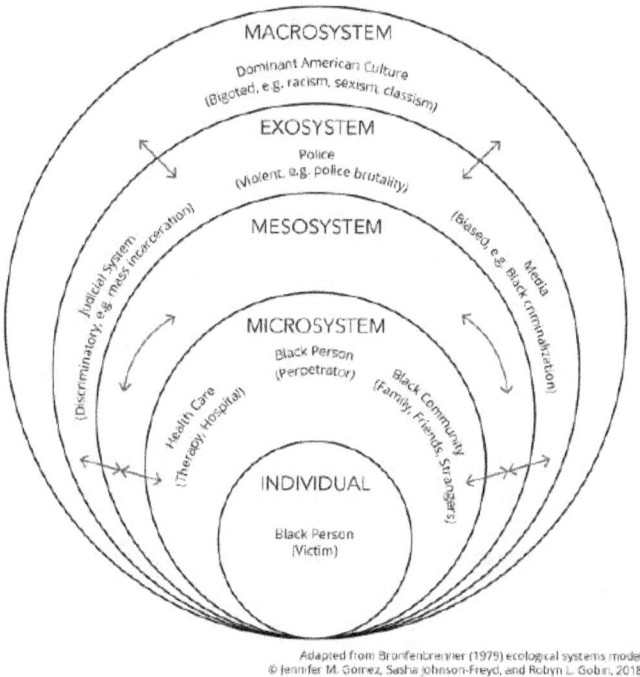

Adapted from Bronfenbrenner (1979) ecological systems model
© Jennifer M. Gómez, Sasha Johnson-Freyd, and Robyn L. Gobin, 2018

CBTT does not assume that all underrepresented groups are the same, but rather recognizes the between-group and within group differences. CBTT also does not imply higher prevalence of trauma in underrepresented groups and recognizes that within-group trauma occurs both in minority groups and majority groups (Gomez, 2019). CBTT, informed by intersectionality of identities, focuses on the within-group trauma and highlights cultural betrayal as a contributing factor to trauma outcomes (Gomez, 2019). Please see Figure 2 for a visual depiction of CBTT.

Figure 2

Cultural Betrayal Trauma Theory

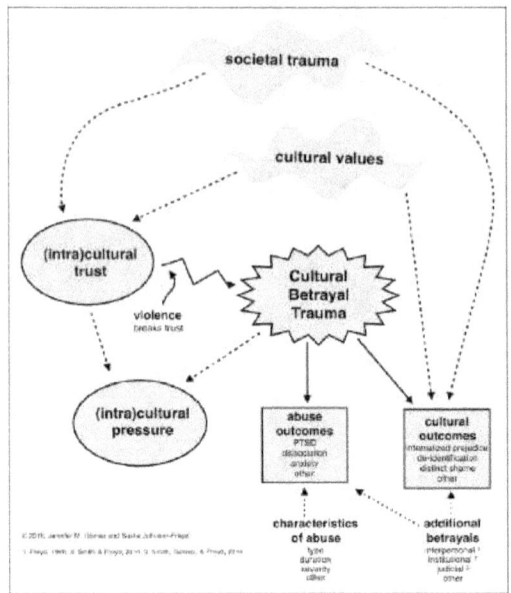

Gomez (2017) theorized that CBTT "contextualizes trauma in interpersonal relationships with trust and/or dependency which creates unique vulnerability to traumatic betrayal" (p.6). In 2019, Gomez found that Black American college students, 47 students enrolled in predominately white university, the "ethno-cultural betrayal trauma predicted posttraumatic stress symptoms" and "posttraumatic (intra)cultural pressure was linked to dissociation" (p. 11). Gomez (2017; 2018; 2019) recognized the need for larger scale studies and studies to measure the adaptability of the theory in different social and cultural contexts specifically in international contexts.

Processing Sexual Trauma

According to Breslouer (2022), healing from traumatic experiences requires taking the memory fragments of the experience and reconstructing the meaning associated with it. In other words, healing is a process of constructing the meaning of the traumatic experience (Breslouer, 2022). Notably, trauma can be triggered, and grief and suffering may result, despite how much time passes after the violence occurred. Lebowitz et al. (1993) highlighted three stages of recovery from trauma based on the empowerment of the victim. In the first stage, victims' primary focus is on developing concrete safety plans and connection to social services to gain a sense of safety and containment. According to the Sexual Assault Support Services (SASS; 2022), this stage is the acute stage of trauma involving the highest sense of fear which may start during the assault and last for several weeks or longer. In the second stage, victims experience remembrance, integration, and mourning that is focused on deep exploration of the traumatic experience (Lebowitz et al., 1993) and involves active uncovering of the trauma. In the third stage victims reconnect with others and integrate the traumatic experience (Lebowitz et al., 1993). In the third stage, the traumatic experience does not intrude on the daily tasks of the survivor and disclosures to family and others may occur (Lebowitz et al., 1993). During this third stage, survivors are able to go through their daily routines without reliving the memories related to the sexual violence (SASS, 2022).

  The journey towards healing after an experience of sexual violence has the potential to be a multifaceted challenge (e.g., Campbell et al., 2009; Wuest et al., 2007). Healing from traumatic experiences should be understood as a focus on the holistic wellbeing through highlighting the strength of the individual rather than placing an emphasis on becoming symptom free (Dahlgren et al., 2020). The Substance Abuse and Mental Health Services Administration (SAMSA, 2014) encourages trauma-based service-providing organizations to incorporate not only trauma-focused assessment and interventions but also work towards ensuring the six principles of creating a safe environment for survivors of trauma: 1) safety; 2) trustworthiness and transparency; 3) peer support; 4) collaboration and mutuality; 5) empowerment, voices and choices; and 6) cultural, historical, and gender issues. Addressing cultural norms and stereotypes that are integral to how a survivor of traumatic experiences interprets and creates meaning is essential in providing trauma-informed care (SAMSA, 2014). Incorporating cultural healing practices and historical trauma in the policies and services available to survivors will assist their journey of processing the experience of sexual violence (SAMSA, 2014). Furthermore, Ginwright (2018) proposes a shift from trauma-informed care to healing-centered care in which practitioners intentionally incorporate the holistic wellbeing of the survivor in their engagement with the individual. Healing-centered care is a strength-based approach that emphasizes the role of culture, spirituality, and collective survival into an individual's journey of surviving from sexual trauma (Ginwright, 2018).

Relationship to Perpetrator

Factors affecting the journey of surviving sexual trauma include situations related to the sexual violence or the relationship between the survivor and perpetrator prior to violence (Freedman & Enrght, 1996; Saint & Sinko, 2019). Researchers found that relationships including incest, child abuse, and date rape, could add to the challenges of processing sexually violent experiences (Saint & Sinko, 2019). Pain and hurt can be deeper when victims perceive betrayal and breaking of the loyalty and trust of the relationship that existed prior to the event (Freedman & Enrght, 1996; Saint & Sinko, 2019). As a result, survivors of incest may be subjected to a higher level of psychological distress than survivors who had no familial relationship with their perpetrator(s) (Freedman & Enright, 1996). The same study showed, however, that by engaging in interventions, survivors can heal from and process their suffering. Similarly, other studies also indicated that distress and/or healing after sexual violence is independent of the relationship between the survivor and perpetrator prior to the sexual violence (Campbell et al., 2009; Freedman & Enright, 2017).

Resiliency Skills

Domhardt et al. (2015) conceptualized resilience as a skill of "adaptive functioning and/or the absence of psychological disorders" (p. 477) following a traumatic experience. Multiple studies have been conducted with the aim of exploring specific interventions and systems that contribute to the journey of surviving after experiencing sexual violence (Campbell et al., 2009; Durà-Vilà et al., 2013; Maxwell et al., 2020; Newsom & Myers-Bowman, 2017; Saint & Sinko, 2019; Sinko et al., 2021; Swanson & Szymanski, 2020). Some studies found resiliency skills to be related to positive posttraumatic growth (e.g., Campbell et al., 2009; Saint & Sinko, 2019). For instance, a study conducted among 206 women in which 78% and 76% identified as Caucasian and heterosexual respectively, revealed that perceived hope and self-compassion were positively related to growth-oriented outcomes during the surviving process (Saint & Sinko, 2019). Relearned coping skills, resiliency skills, hope, and self-compassion were also found to be related to post-traumatic growth (Campbell et al., 2009; Saint & Sinko, 2019). Positive coping strategies such as expressing and processing emotions, asking for help, and meditation were found to be associated with lowered levels of mental health problems (Durà-Vilà et al., 2013; Saint & Sinko, 2019; Swanson & Szymanski, 2020). In a study focusing on the #MeToo movement, specifically interviewed 16 predominantly White adults (12 women, 2 genderqueer/nonconforming, and 1 man & genderqueer) engaged in activism and found that optimism and positive thinking tendencies were associated with faster recovery from sexual trauma (Swanson & Szymanski, 2020).

In 2017, Newsom and Myers-Bowman conducted a phenomenological study on the resiliency skills associated with the survival journey of female sexual violence survivors. The results revealed that self-awareness — consciousness of the internal dialogue — was one of the sources of resilience. In addition, reclaiming personal power and letting go of negative emotions and thoughts were associated with resilience. Participants with more resiliency skills were found to have better mental health outcomes that indicate their positive engagement in their surviving journey (Newsom & Myers-Bowman, 2017). In another study conducted among women survivors of gender-based violence (including sexual abuse), reconnecting with self and gaining control were associated with healing from traumatic experiences (Sinko et al., 2021). As a result, engagement in the process of surviving from sexual trauma could be through reclaiming a sense of lost power and control because of the sexual violence (Maxwell et al., 2020). In searching for the best strategies to help them to regain control, survivors may also choose to engage in nontraditional outlets instead of, for example, engaging in medical or mental health therapy (Maxwell et al., 2020). For instance, Maxwell et al. (2020) reported that women survivors of sexual trauma chose cathartic tattoos to intentionally turn away from the traditional health services that did not meet their needs.

Durà-Vilà et al. (2013) conducted a study among five Spanish and other nationality nuns, and found survivors of sexual trauma revealed community acceptance, spiritual integration, and posttraumatic growth (forgiveness of abusers and awareness of human nature) as stages of the healing journey. In these stages, spiritual transformation was found to be a significant contributor to posttraumatic growth (Durà-Vilà et al., 2013). Few studies, however, were specifically designed to voice the experience of survivors in underrepresented racial, sexual, gender, and ability groups by addressing the role of culture in their journey of processing sexual violence. To ensure the implementation of a holistic approach to processing sexual trauma, studies that address the role of intra- and intercultural solidarity among survivors of sexual violence will be valuable (Gomez, 2019).

Advocacy

Self-empowering activities such as participating in self and group advocacy as well as attempts to connect with others are factors positively related to healing from sexual trauma (Swanson & Szymanski, 2020). The study by Swanson and Szymanski (2020) found that respondents who participated in the #MeToo advocacy movement were able to notice a shift from shame and silence to building relationships, validation, and support. In this study, feeling heard, acknowledged, and supported in a network created through the advocacy journey were positively correlated with the survival process following sexual trauma (Swanson & Szymanski, 2020). However, the #MeToo movement has been criticized for not highlighting the unique experiences of women of color in relation to sexual violence (Leung & Williams, 2019; Onwuachi-Willig, 2018). For instance, the essay by Onwuachi-Willig (2018) argued that the role women of color play in advocacy against workplace sexual violence needs to be emphasized. The #MeToo movement also highlights the heightened vulnerability of women of color in experiencing as well as reporting sexual violence (Onwuachi-Willig, 2018). Leung and Williams (2019) also reiterated the role of race-based stereotypes in highlighting the voices of women of color, despite the fact that pioneers of the #MeToo movement were Black women who advocated for justice before the movement began.

Although women of color pioneered the advocacy efforts towards justice for sexual violence, some are hesitant to speak their truth out of fear -- for themselves and their community -- of possible repercussions from speaking up (Kagal et al., 2019). Kagal et al. (2019) stated that some women of color decided not to engage in the conversation of the #MeToo movement fearing that their community would be judged if they were to speak about their experience involving sexual violence. This argument is similar to the CBTT in emphasizing the role of intracultural pressure and role of an intercultural trust that impact decisions to report sexual violence as well as the healing journey (Gomez, 2018; 2019).

Social Connection

Social connection is another significant factor related to healing from sexual trauma (Ringland, 2017; Sinko et al., 2021). Studies have identified that negative social connections or simply lacking social connections may result in more negative consequences of sexual violence (Ginwright, 2018; Gomez & Gobin, 2019; Saint & Sinko, 2019; Swanson & Szymanski, 2020). For some, social connection is expressed through community acceptance and working to gain the trust and recognition of those around them (Durà-Vilà et al., 2013). As a result, survivors' healing is connected to their perception of feeling valued within their own community. Researchers reported that social connection and networking among survivors of sexual violence was found to be a strong contributor to feeling validated (Swanson & Szymanski, 2020; Sinko et al., 2021). Both studies highlight the significance of collective healing as survivors engage in a movement and find their voices. Other studies emphasize the role of culture as a central concept in the collective journey of surviving (Ginwright, 2018; Gomez & Gobin, 2019). Barriers to connecting with others and achieving the desired level of social connection include fear of judgement and vulnerability (Sinko et al., 2021).

Justice

Justice is another factor associated with the surviving journey of survivors of sexual trauma (Ringland, 2017; Saint & Sinko, 2019). Victims of sexual violence may have different interpretations of what justice means to them. For instance, Ringland (2017) reported that indigenous justice — healing rather than restorative justice — allows individuals to regain balance and heal from traumatic experiences they encountered. Therefore, the process of healing for indigenous survivors of sexual violence could involve reconnecting with themselves by embracing their indigenous values separate from their engagement with the justice system (Ringland, 2017). Swanson and Szymanski (2020) also indicated that the perception of justice was enhanced by survivor's involvement in advocacy that contributed to their improved mental health outcomes. Although studies show perceived justice is associated with positive mental health outcomes (Campbell et al., 2009), unpleasant experiences with the justice system could negatively impact survivors of sexual violence (Saint & Sinko, 2019). A study conducted by Saint and Sinko (2019) highlighted the victim blaming and secondary trauma experienced by some survivors by the justice system. Overall, the perceived justice gained through the legal system and the way the survivor is treated after the violence were found to be associated with survivors' feelings of being validated and supported (Saint & Sinko, 2019).

Forgiveness

Another factor contributing to the process of surviving from sexual trauma is forgiveness (e.g., Enright & Rique, 2004; Prieto-Ursúa, 2021; Tracy, 1999). Forgiveness is a complex concept that involves intrapersonal, dyadic interpersonal, and social and political interpersonal processes (Worthington, 2005). Forgiveness can be a process dealt with solely by the survivor, or it may include the offender and others directly or indirectly involved in the transgression; the aim is repentance and/or reconciliation, without interfering in the need for and process of justice (Enright & Rique, 2004; Prieto-Ursúa, 2021). The general consensus on the importance of forgiveness as a formal clinical or informal intervention to heal from sexual trauma means that, as a tool, survivors of sexual trauma could choose to utilize forgiveness as part of their healing process (James, 2018; Prieto-Ursúa, 2021). However, when proposing forgiveness, careful consideration must be given regarding what forgiveness is and what the process might entail (Prieto-Ursúa, 2021). Tracy (1999) states that forgiveness models that eliminate the possibility of consequences for the actions of the perpetrators can be damaging for survivors of sexual violence. As a result, it is important to emphasize that forgiveness does not mean denying or ignoring survivors' feelings of hurt or excusing the actions of the perpetrator (Freedman & Enright, 2017).

Similarly, forgiveness interventions need to differentiate unforgiveness, forgiveness, and reconciliation (Enright & Rique, 2004; Freedman & Enright, 1996, 2017; Prieto-Ursúa, 2021). The ability to differentiate these concepts in terms of thinking, emotion, and behaviors allows individuals to intentionally integrate forgiveness in their journey of surviving (Freedman & Enright, 1996). Safer (2010) stated that "there is no objective scale for weighing crime of the heart" (p.185) indicating that forgiving and unforgiving is the decision of the beholder. Survivors of sexual trauma may decide to "unforgive" the sexual violence that happened to them, while nevertheless working on accepting that the event has happened (Safer, 2010). Regardless, the choice and the decision process involving forgiveness can be empowering to the survivors of sexual trauma.

Worthington (2005) indicated that the benefits of forgiveness can be associated with areas of physical, mental, relational, and spiritual health, although forgiveness is not the sole contributor of wellbeing in these areas. Several studies have measured the therapeutic benefits of forgiveness (Durà-Vilà et al., 2013; Gildea, 2020; Ha et al., 2019; Hemma et al., 2018; James, 2018; Walton, 2005). In a study of therapeutic intervention incorporating forgiveness, Hemma et al. (2018), found that sexual trauma survivors showed a remarkable improvement in negative mental health symptoms and wellbeing. James (2018), in a phenomenological study among six female date rape survivors (four Caucasian and two African American), also reported that forgiveness was beneficial to letting go of the hurt and anger, empowering the survivor, and helping the survivor show empathy to others. These benefits of forgiveness were associated with positive mental health outcomes for these women (James, 2018).

In 2005, Walton identified a forgiveness model that aimed at helping survivors of sexual abuse. This model emphasized the use of apology and contrition as a framework for therapy and involved the imagination of an apology through a miracle question and an "apology on behalf of" technique. The implementation of this forgiveness model benefitted survivors through empowerment and promoting personal growth, allowing clients to make decisions related to relational or judicial forgiveness (Walton, 2005).

In an autoethnographic study, Gildea (2020) focused on the use of poetry as a forgiveness tool, revealing that forgiveness was facilitated by the art of poetry which then contributed positively to the journey of healing of the survivor. Similarly, in a study conducted among South Korean sexual survivors, Ha et al. (2019), reported that forgiveness writing therapy was associated with decreased symptoms of shame and depression as well as an increased level of post-traumatic growth. This study highlighted that self-forgiveness and forgiveness of the situation can have positive implications rather than the forgiveness of others. However, another study conducted among undergraduate students revealed that the combined efforts of forgiveness of self, others and the situation served as mediators to PTSD symptoms and hostility (Snyder & Heinze, 2005).

In their study of nuns who survived sexual trauma, Durà-Vilà et al. (2013) indicated that forgiving the perpetrators was an important part of posttraumatic growth. The study showed that faith, spirituality, and community acceptance played a significant role for survivors in choosing to forgive their perpetrators.

Forgiveness could extend into having mercy and developing goodwill towards perpetrators by enabling sexual trauma survivors to see their offenders as humans who deserve respect despite their actions (Freedman & Enright, 2017). This shows that forgiveness can focus on more than letting go of anger and increasing self-esteem. Forgiveness was also found to make a significant contribution to the journey of healing for survivors of the deep wounds associated with sexual violence (Freedman & Enright, 1996). Forgiveness therapy allowed women survivors of incest to choose a moral response to hurt, which contributed to feeling empowered and experiencing a decrease in negative psychological outcomes (Freedman & Enright, 1996).

Although several studies have shown the relevance and the possibility of forgiving both the situation and the perpetrator, some therapists prefer to focus on self-forgiveness in their intervention (Davies, 2020). The study by Davies (2020) indicated that the emphasis in their psychoanalytic work with clients is mainly "…focused on helping each of my patients to forgive not the perpetrator of their abuse, but rather themselves" (p.37). The differences in the approaches of therapists and/or intervention programs in focusing on one or all aspects of forgiveness could influence the role of forgiveness in the journey of healing for survivors. Despite the research foundation on the importance of forgiveness to the journey of healing from sexual violence, healing can happen in its absence, as evident in the aforementioned studies focused on justice, social connection, advocacy, resiliency skills, and relationship with the perpetrator.

Socioeconomic and Cultural Background

Socioeconomic and cultural background associated with both the victim and the perpetrator are also related to the journey of healing for the survivor, and studies have found higher levels of mental health issues in sexual violence victims from underrepresented ethnic groups (Campbell et al., 2009; Ginwright, 2018; Gomez & Gobin, 2020). Specifically, Gomez (2016; 2019) and Gomez and Gobin (2020) proposed that the cultural betrayal theory of trauma plays a part in the push and pull that victims of sexual violence feel. The studies further explained that victims may choose to protect the perpetrator against the dominant systems that have historically oppressed underrepresented groups versus seeking justice for themselves to heal from their wounds caused by the sexual violence (Gomez, 2016, 2019; Gomez & Gobin, 2020). Two relevant lines of inquiry are how survivors of sexual violence in underrepresented ethnic groups engage in a process of healing while holding onto their cultural values; and whether cultural betrayal plays a part in survivors' process in other underrepresented groups such as sexual and gender minorities.

Summary of the Conceptual Framework

Most studies on the impacts of sexual violence have not focused on the process of healing (Campbell et al., 2009; Freedman & Enrght, 1996; Saint & Sinko, 2019; Wuest et al., 2007). The one exception, a study by Swanson and Szymanski (2020), investigated the healing process from sexual trauma in relation to survivors' engagement in advocacy and the #MeToo movement. This current study focused on the experience and process of healing that helped identify trauma responses that have contributed to the journey of survivors after an experience of sexual trauma through the lens of cultural considerations that impacted this healing journey.

To understand the holistic process of surviving sexual trauma, this study focused on the specific experiences and process of the integration stage of trauma recovery as well as factors that led to this integration stage. On forgiveness, most studies that include forgiveness report its relevance to improving the mental health of survivors of sexual violence and focus on applying and evaluating a forgiveness therapy or an intervention through measuring symptoms experienced by the survivors of sexual violence (e.g., Freedman & Enright, 2017; Ha et al., 2019; James, 2018; Mayers-Bowman, 2017; Newsom & Myers-Bowman, 2017; Prieto-Ursúa, 2021). Few studies address the complex nature of forgiveness and how it unfolds across time. Learning about the specific process of each stage of trauma responses and the role of other additional factors intersecting with the process provide additional information to understanding the holistic process of healing from sexual trauma.

Statement of the problem

The voices of survivors of sexual violence and trauma as they navigate the role of intracultural and intercultural factors in their journey provide a knowledge base for the services intended to address the mental and physical health needs of survivors. Honoring these voices, specifically of those who identify with underrepresented groups, enable professionals to assist individuals in navigating their journey as they create meaning within their context and positionality. To facilitate the positive progression towards a transformative view of survivors, it is important to move beyond the descriptions of the experience of the sexual violence and trauma to generate a framework to help guide future practice and research. This framework assists in serving survivors of sexual trauma in clinical and educational contexts.

The development of a framework to portray the experience and process of healing from sexual trauma was best achieved through a qualitative approach. This approach enables researchers to follow the direction of the participants as guides to interpreting the meaning of experiences being reported; through this process, researchers then develop and transform their own views (Creswell & Poth, 2018). It was important to learn and explore the movement within the process of learning and owning interventions such as forgiveness and spirituality (Durà-Vilà et al., 2013), therapeutic interventions (Freedman & Enright, 2017), poetry (Gildea, 2020), or advocacy and connection (Swanson & Szymanski, 2020); including the stuck points individuals experienced during the process of surviving sexual trauma. Moreover, for survivors whose journey involved unforgiveness, learning about the self-initiated individual and/or cultural healing strategies, through the lens of cultural betrayal trauma theory, adds to what is known about the process of surviving sexual violence.

Understanding the process and experience of surviving a sexual trauma required an in-depth exploration of the meaning participants gave to what the process represented to them. As individuals discovered their reality, they created a movement that showed the phases of processing a sexual trauma. Grounded theory allows recognition and focus on the flow of these phases of processing sexual trauma as individuals created meaning from their experience (Creswell & Poth, 2018). Through constructivist grounded theory, this dissertation aimed to develop a theory that provides guidance to better understand the process of surviving sexual trauma for those who identify as members of underrepresented groups based on the knowledge co-constructed on the experience of survivors. This study intended to answer the following question: What is the experience and process of underrepresented groups surviving sexual trauma? The goal was to inform ways of enhancing mental and physical health through holistic intervention for survivors of sexual trauma based on what has worked for them thus far.

CHAPTER 2: METHODOLOGY

Qualitative inquiry allows researchers to implement an interpretative naturalistic approach that helps make the experiences of individuals visible (Creswell & Poth, 2018). In qualitative research, the researcher studies the participants in their natural settings, and attempts to make sense of participants' experiences based on the meaning people bring to them (Creswell & Poth, 2018). The journey of processing a traumatic experience is unique to each individual survivor and qualitative inquiry enables researchers to represent these different voices.

Among the factors that influence the process of surviving, healing, and making meaning of surviving from sexual violence are the identities an individual holds in their community(ies) (Gomez, 2016; 2019; Gomez & Gobin, 2020). For instance, identities related to race, class, gender, disability, employment, etc. could speak to the power participants hold in a position of privilege (unearned or taken for granted) and/or oppression (Denzin, 2017). Working from a critical stance and practicing reflexivity enables researchers to develop methodological self-awareness in which researchers recognize their own power as they co-construct knowledge with participants from diverse identities (Charmaz, 2017).

This dissertation utilized a qualitative approach to study how various identities intersect with the process of experiencing sexual trauma, and ultimately how survivors view their world after the traumatic experience. As individuals reflect on their experience of surviving from sexual trauma, their interpretation and meaning-making of the experience of surviving could be influenced by their position historically, socially, culturally, and contextually (Creswell & Poth, 2018). Because of their positionality, the meaning individuals give to the world as well as their interaction with it is subjective; individuals who have gone through similar events may have different views and interpretations of the experience and individually shaped emotional, cognitive, and behavioral reactions. Qualitative approaches enable the researcher to be guided by the data in the field and adjust the research protocols in response to their interaction with the participants, adapting, for example, the data collection strategies and even the research questions (Creswell & Poth, 2018). This inductive/bottom-up approach emphasizes learning from participants' experience and uses the data to develop a framework/theory that helps guide practices.

In this qualitative inquiry, I used Charmaz's (2006) constructivist grounded theory and Clarke's (2003) situational analysis to guide engagement with participants, data collection, analysis, and interpretation. Below I describe the interpretive frameworks and methods to guide the process of co-constructing knowledge related to the experience and process of surviving from sexual trauma for individuals identifying as members of underrepresented groups.

Interpretive Framework

Creswell and Poth (2018) stated that qualitative researchers need to choose a framework/paradigm to help them understand and articulate the overall process of the research. Interpretive frameworks allow qualitative researchers to situate their philosophical assumptions into their approach of practice. In this study, I used critical theory and social constructivism as interpretive frameworks. In alignment with the social constructivism interpretive framework (Creswell & Poth, 2018), I recognize that world views are constructed through the interaction of the individual with their social and historical context, resulting in multiple and complex meanings and views. Moreover, I used critical qualitative inquiry (Creswell & Poth, 2018) to reflect on the role of my own power and privilege while interacting with study participants. In addition, I interpreted participants' identities, and its intersectionality with their journey of surviving from sexual trauma, though the lens of critical theory by recognizing the role of the power and positionality of participants as they give meaning to their traumatic experience.

Critical qualitative inquiry

Operating from a critical stance allows researchers to examine the social, historical, and contextual factors that shape our world view (Creswell & Poth, 2018). The power, privilege, and/or oppressions associated with race, class, gender, disability, etc. can shape the positionality of individuals in their social situation (Creswell & Poth, 2018). The positionality associated with their identities and social situations can, in turn, shape the experience and process of survivors of sexual trauma in underrepresented groups, due to social, cultural, and historical factors (Gomez, 2018, 2019). In addition, Creswell and Poth (2018) stated that critical qualitative researchers engage in reflexivity to recognize their power and role as they enter a dialogue with their participants with the aim of constructing a theory; a theory that allows them to interpret a social action.

Rooted in a human rights agenda, critical inquiry seeks a transformative paradigm and challenges the existing system and culture related to inequalities and injustices based on the situatedness of individuals in their social context (Denzin, 2017). A critical qualitative inquiry can give voice to the daily experiences related to social justice (Denzin, 2017) as well as recognize the existence of multiple realities within the context of social justice (Koro-Ljungberg & Cannella, 2017). Denzin (2017) stated that critical qualitative inquiry researchers are ethically responsible to center the voices of the participants, indicate areas for change and activism, and model change as they engage with their participants.

In this study, I recognize that the journey of surviving from sexual trauma for individuals in underrepresented groups intersects with their social, cultural, and historical context. I openly recognize my positionality in my own social contexts and the power I held while I interacted with participants for this study. As I engaged in the process of co-constructing knowledge, using critical qualitative inquiry helped me to be curious about and recognize multiple interpretations of participants' experience and the process of their journey with sexual trauma, as influenced by their situatedness and social context. The role of power and privilege was also confirmed in interviews with study participants as well as during the two rounds of data analysis; that is, participants noted the different power and privileges they held or did not hold as they interpreted their experience of sexual violence. I also witnessed participants' perceptions of their aggressor's power and privilege in the world.

Social constructivism

Social constructivism proposes that "meanings are negotiated socially and historically...[meanings] are not simply imprinted on individuals but are formed through interaction with others" (Creswell & Poth, 2018, p. 24). This implies that individuals form their reality, perspectives, and meanings based on interactions with events and social and historical situations. Social constructivism argues that meanings are made through discussions and/or interactions with others, and that researchers need to actively listen to the content and language in participants' expressions (Creswell & Poth, 2018). Charmaz (2006), in her constructivist grounded theory, stated that knowledge created during qualitative inquiry is co-constructed between the researcher and the participants. Designing studies from a social constructivist framework allows participants to construct their meaning and tell their story (Charmaz, 2006; Creswell & Poth, 2018). In practice, this requires researchers to pose broader and general questions and then follow the participants' lead as they construct the meaning of their process of surviving sexual trauma (Creswell & Poth, 2018). Accordingly, during the two rounds of interviews with the participants, I asked general semi-structured guiding questions and followed up with their initial disclosures. I also used paraphrases and clarifying questions to confirm their viewpoints in their meaning-making process. Charmaz (2006) stated that constructivist grounded theory and its principles and practices allow researchers to capture the movement within an experience and see the participants' world from the inside out. In this study, I engaged in the co-construction of multiple realities with each participant that enabled me to develop themes that represent the experience and process of their journey following sexual violence. In this dissertation study, I used Charmaz (2006)'s constructivist grounded theory and Clarke's (2003) situational analysis to guide the data collection, formulation, and analysis.

Charmaz's constructivist grounded theory. In its foundation, grounded theory emphasized the role of interaction and meaning making in understanding human problems, and was intended to answer "what", "how" and "why" questions related to the situation under study (Uri, 2015). Grounded theory presented new ways of looking at knowledge and data by introducing simultaneous, continuous, and comparative interaction with the data at each stage of the research process, so a theory could be developed using the data that originated from the field (Charmaz, 2006; 2017). Charmaz (2006, 2017) argued that using the constructivist grounded theory approach and principles requires researchers to be reflective and be methodologically self-conscious. The process of reflectivity and methodological self-awareness enables the researcher to have a critical stance whereby they explicitly reflect on their situatedness in their social context as they interpret the positionality of their participants (Charmaz, 2017).

As a result, I asked questions about what contributed to healing and obstacles to healing, how these participant experiences were connected, and why participants made certain decisions as they engaged in the process of healing from sexual trauma. I used a researcher journal and memoing to increase my methodological awareness. I took notes on my experience following the interviews with participants and reflected on my reactions as I transcribed and coded the interviews. I also consulted with my inquiry auditor during the initial and focused coding processes to help ground my observations based on the data.

The process of co-constructing knowledge between the researcher and participants, and mapping situations involving the social factors in the participants' experience and process, creates the opportunity to build theory through inductive approaches (Creswell & Poth, 2018). Inductive approaches enable researchers to co-construct knowledge through open-ended and emergent methods that cultivate critical stances. Accordingly, in this study, open coding was done to identify emerging participants' experience and build a theory about the survival journey following sexual violence. This is consistent with Charmaz (2020), who suggested to constructivist researchers on the need to practice reflexivity throughout their study and work towards methodological self-awareness to be able to hold a critical stance.

Charmaz's (2006) constructivist approach to grounded theory has the following assumptions: "(1) reality is multiple, processual, and constructed—but constructed under particular conditions; (2) the research process emerges from interaction; (3) it takes into account the researcher's positionality, as well as that of the research participants; and (4) the researcher and researched co-construct the data—data are a product of the research process, not simply observed objects of it" (Charmaz, 2006, p. 402). In this study, the philosophical assumptions were formulated in line with those of Charmaz's constructivist grounded theory. Participants were asked general guiding questions during both interviews to allow them to expand on their reality about the events leading up to, during, and following the sexual violence experience. As they disclosed particular events, views, and perceptions, I asked follow-up questions intended to allow each participant to elaborate on what is true to them. Data were then constructed through these guiding and clarifying questions and statements.

Grounded theory and situational analysis. Based on the assumptions of Charmaz's constructivist grounded theory, Clarke (2005) developed situational analysis to portray the situatedness and positionality within contexts by constructing maps of relatedness among actors and contexts. Situational analysis allows researchers to draw theory through inductive and abductive reasoning by mapping what was known through prolonged engagement with participants (Clarke, 2009; Uri, 2015). During the two rounds of analyses, mapping the positionality within their social and historical context helped me to understand how sexual trauma survivors navigated their journey in relation to power associated with their identities and its intersection.

Situational analysis involves developing three kinds of maps (Clarke, 2003; 2009): 1) situational maps; 2) social worlds/arenas; and 3) positional maps. Situational maps are described as a process to "lay out the major human, nonhuman, discursive, and other elements in the research situation of inquiry and provoke analysis of relations among them" (Clarke, 2009, p. 210). Clarke stated that situational maps are intended to capture the "messy complexities" that occur among the actors and of the situation in the research. I used situational analysis to map the emerging themes based on the data co-constructed in the field with the participants. The situational map is intended to be done and redone throughout the study to allow the researcher to start making relationships among and between actors and actants within the situation (Clarke, 2003). This was true in my experience as well. I developed 15 versions of situational maps to identify the socio-cultural, contextual and identity-based factors that impacted participants' journey following sexual violence. Clarke (2003) indicated that researchers will know a "good enough" situational map indicating relations of all involved actors in a situation when they reach saturation. In the final version of the conceptual map, the map feels complete and full representation of all the experiences and processes have emerged based on the participants' experiences.

Ontology

The meaning, process, and experience of surviving a sexual trauma is subjective based on the interaction of each survivor with their intra and intercultural contexts. Thus, what is real, and the meaning given to that reality, is different for each individual. In constructivist approaches, researchers recognize and embrace the existence of multiple realities (Charmaz, 2006; Creswell & Poth, 2018) and pure objectivity of the researcher is impossible. Constructivist approaches recognize that reality is constructed through the engagement of the person with the world, and that language serves as a main tool for making sense of the world (Duffy & Chenail, 2008). Therefore, researchers report multiple realities that are organized in multiple themes representing the voices of different individuals and showing different perspectives (Creswell & Poth, 2018).

As a researcher, in line with the propositions of the social constructivism and critical inquiry interpretive frameworks, I believe participants construct meaning from their experience through interaction with their social, cultural, and historical environments. This includes the interaction of the researcher and the participant creating the opportunity for the co-construction of knowledge. Therefore, in this research on the experience and process of surviving sexual trauma, I recognized that participants' meanings were multiple and shaped by their social, cultural, and historical experiences. In addition, what they considered to have contributed to their process of surviving sexual trauma depended on their experiences and interactions with their social and historical environment including the aggressor. As evident in the emerging experiences and processes, participants' positionality and power also influenced how they navigated their journey of surviving sexual trauma. Participants' decisions to seek justice, personal trauma responses, disclosures and other additional parts of their experience were shaped by their sociocultural contexts and power and privilege associated with their intersecting identities. This fact has resulted in the existence of multiple realities expressed through perspectives and words representing these experiences. I organized multiple themes derived from these realities learned from each individual participant and created a theory to explain the experience and process of surviving from sexual trauma.

Epistemology

The decisions regarding what constitutes knowledge, the relationship between the knowers and the would-be knowers, and how knowledge is known constitute the concept of epistemology (Creswell & Poth, 2018). In a constructivist interpretive framework, "knowledge is not a thing-in-itself, but rather provides a blueprint for human adaptation and movement through the world" (Duffy & Chenail, 2008, p. 29). Charmaz (2006) argues that knowledge is gained through the interaction of the participants and the researcher. The researcher discovers and co-constructs knowledge as a result of interacting with participants. Charmaz's constructivist approach recognizes the collaborative nature of knowing through prolonged engagement of the learner with the knower. In this case, knowledge is co-created through the interaction between the participant and the researcher as participants respond to the research questions concerning the process and experience involving a social action i.e., sexual trauma.

I used paraphrases and clarifying questions during the interview as I co-constructed the knowledge regarding participants' experience following sexual violence. I recognized that prolonged engagement with participants during the data collection and analysis would help minimize the distance between the research participants and myself. To this end, I conducted two interviews with each participant, transcribed the interviews and reviewed the transcripts, coded each transcript, and identified each quote that supported the themes emerging based on participants' experiences. Language -- both verbal (words expressed by participants) and non-verbal communications (such as facial expressions, tone of voice, emphasis on expressions, gestures, etc.) -- served a key role in co-constructing knowledge with participants. Therefore, the co-construction of knowledge between myself and my participants was facilitated by the language I used during my interaction with the participants and the data itself. In addition, I added the nonverbal expressions of participants such as silence, laughter, nervous laughter, etc. as I transcribed the interviews. These nonverbal communications were included as part of the analysis, and quotes taken from these transcripts included both verbal and nonverbal language participants used during the interview.

Recognizing the influence of my own identities as an African Black non-US born woman, and my past and present experiences on how I understand and interact with participants, I introduced myself and my intent to conduct this study. During one of the interviews, I found it important that I shared my collectivist culture background and cultural views on masculine sexual behaviors to create a relatable experience for the interviewee. This disclosure did not change the direction of the discussion, although it was helpful for the interviewee to normalize some cultural views that could otherwise have been considered unacceptable.

Collaboration between myself and my participants during the data collection, as well as the analysis process, was paramount to my understanding of the knowledge as perceived by them. As a result, I created semi-structured guiding questions that allowed participants to openly share their views and perspectives and help me learn and co-create meaning about the situation under study. Knowledge or data in this case represented the words and expressions of meanings the participants gave to their own world as interpreted through their positionality based on their identities. In addition to the collaborative knowledge creation process during the interview, I answered any questions participants had about the data analysis process, and shared the newly developed framework with each participant to get their perspectives on how well their knowledge was represented.

Approaching this study through critical theory and social constructivism allowed me to recognize participants' positionality and my own values and role as I interacted with the knowledge co-constructed with my participants as well as implemented ethical decisions to ensure the trustworthiness of the data.

Axiology

In qualitative study, the researcher is recognized as value-laden, and biases are present emanating from the lived experience of the researcher. Creswell and Poth (2018) stated that all researchers bring values into their study. As a qualitative researcher, however, it is important to recognize and disclose values within the study by sharing the researchers' positionality in relation to the context and the content. In a constructivist interpretive framework "what is said and what is not said has ethical importance" (Duffy & Chenail, 2008, p. 29). I am aware that, in addition to what I openly disclosed to participants, the color of my skin and my English accent (for example) communicate my visible identities to my participants.

Charmaz (2017) argues that constructivist grounded theory calls for methodological self-consciousness which in turn requires researcher's reflexivity throughout the study. Methodological self-consciousness requires approaching co-construction of knowledge by developing awareness and explicit recognition of privileges, both unearned and/or taken for granted (Charmaz, 2017). Through reflexivity, researchers examine their and their participants' positionality, power, and subjectivity by analyzing their worldviews, language, and meanings in relation to the study (Charmaz, 2017; 2020). Methodological self-awareness allows researchers to question existing assumptions, and critically examine justices and injustices within the social and historical contexts influencing their world view.

I recognize that my own demographic, social, professional, and historical positions shape my values and thereby my interpretations of the knowledge learned from the participants. I used the assumptions of a constructivist approach combined with critical stance as I continuously reflected on my own personal values and where I am situated in my identities. Therefore, the process of co-construction of knowledge throughout my interaction with my participants was shaped by my values and my positionality. As a result, with each theme and supporting quotes, assisted by my inquiry auditor, I practiced reflexivity and engaged with the data for a significant amount of time to make sure the data were appropriately defined and accurately represented.

Methodology

Grounded theory is a method to "generate or discover a theory" to help us explain the movement within the process of an action (Creswell & Poth, 2018). This allowed me to develop a framework about how survivors process an experience of sexual trauma. I chose grounded theory as a method for this dissertation for two reasons: 1) grounded theory focuses on processes that have phases/steps over time; and 2) grounded theory helps researchers to see the flow of the process (Creswell & Poth, 2018). Processing takes place within the socio-cultural context of the survivor of sexual trauma as time creates the space for individuals to realize what it means for them to heal.

My approach to the grounded theory principles and practices was guided by Charmaz's constructivist approach and I was engaged in the process of enhancing my methodological self-awareness to hold a critical stance. Through the critical theory interpretive framework, I reflected on my identities to recognize my positionality and the related power and privileges as I interacted with the participants. I recognized that my interpretation of the views expressed in the field by participants led to the development of a theory/framework of processing sexual trauma. In addition, I used Clarke's situational analysis to map the relations between and among the actors within the intra- and intercultural contexts of the participants. This situational mapping was helpful in recognizing the sociocultural contexts and socializations that shaped the identities of participants as well as their views on sexual behaviors and trauma.

Below, I explain specific procedures I implemented as I formulated the research questions and the initial sample as well as interacted with the participants during the data collection and analysis.

Research Question

Creswell and Poth (2018) suggest that qualitative researchers develop a single "open-ended, evolving, non-directional, ... [and] overarching" question centered on their research approach to narrow down their study (Creswell & Poth, 2018, p. 137). They asserted that grounded theory studies focus on the "what" of the experience and process related to an action to facilitate the formulation of a theory. Similarly, Tweed and Charmaz (2012) asserted that grounded theory questions are intended to critically examine the subjective interpretation, meaning, pattern, and process of participants' experience in their positionality within their social context. Through the lens of constructivist grounded theory, this study aimed to capture the movement within the experience and process of surviving sexual trauma. This movement happens as individuals create meaning for their healing journey within their intra and intercultural context. As a result, I asked: what is the experience and process of surviving sexual trauma for individuals in underrepresented groups?

Sampling and Participant Selection Procedures

The population for this study were adult survivors of sexual violence from underrepresented groups. As a result, participants aged 20 or above participated in this study with the youngest participant being 21 years old and the oldest 40 years old at the time of the first-round interview. According to Charmaz (2006), in constructing a grounded theory, it is important to start with theoretical sampling to help researchers represent the categories identified within the research topic. As Charmaz (2006) states "initial sampling is where you start..." and "researchers establish sampling criteria by people, cases, situations, and/or settings before entering the field" (p. 100). For a grounded theory study, Guest et al (2006) found that researchers were able to develop a code book with meaningful themes and useful interpretations after conducting six interviews and obtain saturation after twelve interviews. Guided by Guest et al.'s (2006) research outcome, I determined the sample size for the initial sampling of this study to be six participants and I conducted two rounds of interviews with six survivors of sexual violence. Participants were all members of an underrepresented group based on their race, gender identity, sexual orientation, and/or disability status (see Appendix D and Appendix E).

In focus of this study was the movement within the journey of surviving from sexual trauma. This means participants did not need to self-identify as "healed or healing" from sexual trauma, but rather identify themselves as able to engage in the integration stage of trauma recovery and be ready to disclose their experience to a researcher. The requirement of being at the integration stage of trauma recovery was explicitly stated in the participant recruitment email and flyer as *"Identifying as a survivor of adulthood sexual violence and the sexual trauma is no longer intruding on your daily functioning."* Additionally, participants who had not disclosed their experience of sexual violence and trauma prior to their interest in participating in this research were not included. This is because first time disclosure may indicate that the survivor has not had the opportunity to start the process of meaning making; and the participants may not be able to go beyond sharing the event and the aftermath of the event to reflect on what it means to survive the trauma. As a result, the participant recruitment email and flyer incorporated the following eligibility criteria: *"have disclosed your experience to another person prior to participating in this study."*

Due to the sensitivity of the content and the potential of being triggered during the interview process, I followed these ethical consideration guidelines:

1) I prepared a list of resources and mental health services tailored towards sexual trauma (Appendix H).

2) I ensured participants were informed about the local and national resources helping survivors of sexual violence including information about mental health crisis lines. (Two participants refused to take the resources: one is a professional counselor and the second disclosed that they started seeing a therapist following the first-round interview.)

3) If participants were emotional during the interview, I stopped and asked if they wanted to pause, have water and/or time before proceeding, or if they would like to discontinue the discussion. (This only happened with one participant. The participant stated their interest to continue, and the interview was completed without another incident.)

4) I provided participants with my email and cell phone number information and informed them about my openness and availability to call/email/text with questions and referrals for mental health services. I also provided them with an email address my dissertation chair, included in the consent form, for any concerns and questions they may have throughout their participation in this study.

5) I collected participants' emergency contact information (Appendix G) so I could communicate with their emergency contact person in the unlikely event of a crisis involving the participant.

6) Moreover, I had a prior instructor-student relationship with one of the participants during Spring 2021 academic semester. This participant reached out to me to express their interest to participate in this study after seeing the flyer. Given that I: 1) haven't

had any personal and professional relationship with this participant for the past approximately two years and 2) am not currently in any instructor/supervisory/peer/etc... roles with the participant, I accepted their participation in this study. Prior to the interview and during the verbal review process for the informed consent, I informed the participant my dissertation chair's and my committee's association with the UM's Department of Counseling program and the potential for this disclosure to be identified. The participant was in full agreement with these conditions and signed the consent form.

To achieve heterogeneity within this homogenous group of sexual trauma survivors, I looked for diversity in the demographic backgrounds of my participants. Studies indicated that individuals who identify as members of racial, gender, sexual, and ability underrepresented groups experience higher incidents of sexual violence and trauma symptoms (Gomez & Gobin, 2019; Luo et al., 2014; Paquette et al., 2021; Sigurvinsdottir & Ullman, 2016; Whitton et al., 2021). The process of construction of meaning of this traumatic experience is often directed by how the survivors are positioned in their communities. For instance, Gomez and Gobin (2019) indicated that systemic oppression and the meaning Black women give to their and their community members' experience of oppression influence their process of constructing meaning from sexual trauma. Gomez (2005) also noted the role of intra and intercultural connection and meaning in shaping how individuals process sexual trauma.

To ensure the representation of individuals in non-dominant groups, I included participants from a variety of identities, and the six sexual trauma survivors who participated in this study have intersections of multiple underrepresented and privileged identities. Table 1 describes the identities represented in this study.

Table 1

Maximum variation

Identity	Identity group	Number
Race	White	3
	Filipino/Pasifika American	1
	Hispanic white	1
	Asian/ Mixed	1
Disability	Autism/ADHD/panic attacks	1
Sexual orientation	Pansexual	2
	Bisexual/queer	1
	Queer	1
	Sexually oriented towards the female gender	1
	Heteroflexible	1
Gender	Non-binary	3
	Female	1
	Male	1
	Gender expansive	1

Charmaz (2006) indicated that the purpose of theoretical sampling is to "obtain data to help you explicate your categories" (p. 100). Theoretical sampling is related to theory development and not with representativeness of the sample (Charmaz, 2006). When researchers notice that these categories are full, it shows the thickness and richness of the data (Charmaz, 2006). After conducting the first-round and second-round interviews and investigating the themes that emerged based on the data, the data had reached saturation. I determined saturation after recognizing that thick and rich data had been collected from the six participants during the two rounds of interviews, and that no additional themes and processes were emerging based on the data collected.

To recruit participants, I developed a participant recruitment email (Appendix D) explaining the goal of the study, eligibility criteria, and incentives. This email was used to communicate with organizations actively working with sexual trauma survivors and other professional organizations. I also created a flyer (Appendix E) with similar information to be posted around hallways and social media platforms. Both the recruitment email and flyer included my email address and phone number and asked participants to contact me if they were interested in participating in the study. Both were approved by the University of Montana's IRB under #213-22 (Appendix A & B). A twenty-five-dollar Amazon Gift Card incentive were made available for each participant. This incentive for participants was made possible with the Association of Counselor Education and Supervision (ACES)'s Student research award grant that I received for this dissertation study. Gift cards were distributed to each participant prior to the second-round interview.

Initially, I reached out to organizations via the participant recruitment email and/or posted the email on social media platforms when applicable. I also reached out to my professional and personal connections asking them to share the recruitment email with their national and local contacts. Once the flyer was approved, I shared it for easy access and posting around the organizations' physical offices, websites, and social media accounts. The list of organizations and social media platforms I reached out to, as well as the buildings where the flyers were posted, can be found in Appendix I.

When interested participants reached out to me, I asked them to complete a Qualtrics survey asking for demographic information (Appendix F) before being accepted for an interview. This allowed me to check whether all eligibility criteria were met and ensured diversity of participant identities. The demographic question survey included questions about their gender, sexual orientation, race, ability status and the length of time lapsed after the incident involving sexual trauma. Additional questions asked whether participants required disability accommodation and if they experienced sexual violence before the age of 18. The responses to these demographic questions helped to ensure that the maximum variation of identities were included in the study. A total number of 11 sexual trauma survivors expressed interest in participating and six participants met the recruitment criteria.

Once a participant was determined eligible to participate, I contacted them with the means of communication they used to initially contact me to express their interest in the study. In my communication, I specified my availability and options to either meet in person or via Zoom. One participant preferred to meet via Zoom during both the first and second-round interviews, and another participant chose to meet via Zoom during the second-round interview. The remaining interviews were conducted in person.

Before signing their agreement to participate in the study, I verbally reviewed each segment of the consent form (Appendix C) with each participant and had participants complete the emergency contact information form. Once the first round of interviews was concluded, I informed participants that I would reach out for the second-round interview and later on to get their feedback on my findings once I complete both rounds of analyses. All agreed to meet for both interviews and provide their thoughts during the member check. During both rounds of interviews, after I stopped the recording, I asked participants about their experience of participating in the interview and whether they had any feedback for me. At the end of the first-round interview, I shared a copy of the list resources on trauma I had created prior to the interview.

Data Gathering Method

As Charmaz (2006) states "...grounded theory starts as we enter the field where we gather data..." (p. 13) and evolves into theory development. The primary tool for data collection in grounded theory is an interview (Creswell & Poth, 2018) to generate thick and rich data. Beuthin (2014) also noted critical developments in the value placed on interview as a method of data collection for qualitative studies, commenting on the interview's shift from "straightforward method of data collection to a dynamic transformational conversation" (p. 125) with the aim of gathering in dept data about the situation under study. I recognize the value of an interview for the richness of the data and the interaction with participants. I also believe that interviews can be a way of co-constructing meaning together with the participant rather than merely providing a means of exchanging information.

I used a semi-structured interview as a data gathering tool to learn about the experience and process of surviving sexual trauma. The interview was designed to be interactive with participants by asking general guiding questions that allowed them to share the meaning they created, or are creating, regarding their experience and process of surviving sexual trauma. I asked follow-up and clarifying questions as participants disclosed their experience. In this research, data represented the knowledge obtained through the prolonged interaction of the researcher and the participant(s) through the interview. As stated in Charmaz and Belgrave (2018), data is "jointly constructed between the researcher and the participant" (p. 747). In this type of interview data represents bringing the voices of those who would otherwise not be seen or included into an understanding a social phenomenon.

Each interview was planned to last for approximately an hour with a 5–15-minute check-in after the interview questions were completed. The shortest first-round interview time was 47 minutes and the longest was 69 minutes. During the second-round interview, the shortest time was a 28-minute zoom interview (this was partly due to multiple internet interruptions and the participant's inability to describe her experience succinctly without going into detail), and the longest was 62 minutes. During the additional check-in time I: 1) asked participants about how they were feeling and what they needed as we wrapped up the discussion; 2) shared resources and information on mental health services; 3) provided information focusing on sexual trauma if requested by participants; and 4) asked whether they would recommend others to participate in this study. Although this check-in time was neither recorded nor part of the data analysis and interpretation, I took notes of the discussions to support any ethical decisions made after the interview. All participants were willing to be recorded; interviews were video- and audio-recorded on Zoom, and on additional audio recording equipment. No participant expressed need for accommodation except one person who preferred a quiet place for the in-person interview. Data were stored in a secure cloud storage.

Charmaz (2006) stated that questions guiding a grounded theory study shall "create analysis of action and process" (p, 20). In developing the interview guides, I focused on questions that allowed me to see the intra– and interpersonal processes of surviving sexual trauma and learn the actions participants took to facilitate their process. I used the following questions to guide the conversation during my first interview with participants.

1. How would you describe your process of surviving a sexual trauma?
2. Was there a particular moment, or set of events, that really changed the trajectory of your surviving journey? Can you tell me more about that/those?
3. What was something or some things you found especially challenging in your process of healing? What were some things that were especially helpful?
4. Are there moments when your healing has become especially clear to you? What are those?

5. Are there moments when you uncover more work to do, and how do those moments present?

After analyzing the first round of data, second-round interview questions were developed to identify processes that connected the themes that emerged during the first-round analysis as well as fill any gaps and answer any questions that emerged during the first-round data analysis. Below is a list of semi-structured guiding questions I used during the second-round analysis:

1. Thank you for bringing an artifact with you today; can you tell me about it and the meaning it holds in your healing process?
2. What role has time played in your journey after sexual trauma?
3. How do you think your intersecting identities (as a queer/person of color/gender minority/disabled) relate to your responses to sexual trauma?
4. Have you experienced moments of relief from systemic oppression? If so, how are those moments of relief related to or different from your moments of relief from sexual trauma?
5. How did your perpetrator hold power in the world (e.g., as a white male)? Did their power and privilege impact your process of healing?
6. Looking back on your healing journey from where you are now, what meaning do you make of your process?
7. Is there anything we haven't talked about in your healing process that you'd like me to know about?

I asked follow-up questions based on the disclosures of participants as they responded to the second-round questions.

Data Analysis Procedures

Charmaz (2006) defines grounded theory coding as "the pivotal link between collecting data and developing an emergent theory to explain these data" (p. 46). She goes on to say that there are two phases of coding: "(1) an initial phase involving naming each word, line, or segment of data followed by (2) a focused selective phase that uses the most significant or frequent initial codes to sort, synthesize, integrate, and organize large amount of data" (p. 46). I was guided by Charmaz's constructivist grounded theory to code and analyze the data collected from the participants.

At the beginning of each interview, I asked each participant to choose a pseudonym to protect their confidentiality. The recorded data obtained through the interviews was transcribed. I transferred the audio data from each interview to Microsoft Word, reviewed the accuracy of the transcript, and then uploaded each file to NVivo version 12 for the coding process. Each participant's chosen pseudonym was used to name the word file to protect their confidentiality, and was also used in the report writing. Once the transcripts were uploaded on NVivo, I used open coding to develop initial codes. There were 540 initial codes during the first-round analysis. Using focused coding, these 540 initial codes were merged into seven emerging themes and their supporting subcategories, properties, and dimensions. An additional 284 initial codes were identified during the second-round analysis bringing the total number of initial codes to 824. After the second analysis, these 824 codes were merged into five categories.

As suggested by Charmaz (2006), during the initial coding it is important to "remain open, be close to the data, keep the codes simple and precise, preserve actions, and compare data to data" (p. 49). To do so, I used memoing and reflexivity to record my processes as I conducted the initial coding. Specifically, during the initial open coding process, I used word-by-word and line-by-line coding. In this process, I went through each line of the written data and coded actions, processes and experiences that tell the journey of the participants. I then identified the leading categories connected in the voices of the participants. Incidents reported by participants were also identified during the initial coding. These incidents were important for incident-to-incident coding especially in identifying strategies relevant to the process of surviving sexual trauma as recognized by participants. Charmaz (2006) stated that comparing incidents to incidents will help researchers to create themes and patterns that were not able to be identified through line-by-line coding. I used incident-to-incident and comparison coding to identify similarities and differences that helped me gain insights regarding dissimilarities (Charmaz, 2006).

During the second coding phase, I used focused coding, which is used to "synthesize and explain larger segments of data" (Charmaz, 2006, p. 57) after the initial line-by-line coding. Through focused coding, I determined the accuracy and adequacy of the frequent and non-frequent codes identified in the initial phase. As Charmaz (2006) states, focused coding is not a linear process. During this focused coding process, I was able to identify, and correct initial codes missed or coded wrong. In this phase, I moved through the interviews to compare experiences and processes of surviving sexual trauma and reviewed the merging categories, subcategories, properties, and dimensions with my inquiry auditor. When an unexpected or new code emerged, it was recorded, and the data were compared with the previously emerged themes to highlight the new content identified. According to Charmaz (2006), through the process of focused coding, it is possible to recognize "identifying moments" (pp. 59 - 60), which are telling actions and processes shared by many participants of the study. Through comparing data in the focused coding, I was able to find identifying moments that helped create the core of the theory/framework while also recognizing the unique voices represented in the study. The same initial and focused coding procedure was used during the second-round analysis. Moreover, I used axial coding to identify the connections and processes between and among the emerging themes.

Additionally, I used Clarke's situational analysis to create conceptual maps to represent the framework that explained participants' situatedness in their social, cultural, and historical contexts as they navigate their journey following an experience of sexual violence. Situational analysis allows researchers to identify the context and positionality as well as identify the relations that exist between and among the actors and characters of the situation under study (Clarke, 2009). To portray relations, contexts and positionality, Clarke (2003; 2009) suggested mapping of the situation as a way to "open up" the data and portray relations among the actors and characters of the situation. The assumptions of her situational analysis theory are in line with Charmaz's constructivist approach to grounded theory (Clarke, 2009). As a result, I created conceptual maps to represent the framework of the journey following an experience of sexual violence.

Procedures for Establishing Trustworthiness

The design of qualitative research is "fluid and open-ended" (Haverkamp, 2005, p. 147). To achieve rigor in qualitative study, Lincoln and Guba (2007) emphasized methods to assess the internal validity, applicability, replicability/transferability, and neutrality of the data collected. I understand the ethical decisions made in this study are guided by the process in each step of the research. To ensure authentic representation of the voices of the participants, researchers need to develop deep reflexivity and methodological self-consciousness

(Charmaz, 2017; Charmaz & Belgrave, 2018). I used a constructivist approach to data collection which required me to engage in a deeper examination of my privileged or oppressed status, cultural background, and viewpoints as I interacted and co-constructed knowledge with the research participants, and as I analyzed and interpreted the results.

I used the following are the processes to ensure the trustworthiness of the research as well as guide ethical decisions.

Inquiry Audit. As a researcher, I recognize my role and connectedness to this topic and study. My dissertation chair, who has experience in advocacy and counseling working with survivors of sexual trauma, served as my inquiry auditor. She reviewed the emerging focused codes during the first and second-round analyses and the meanings that were assigned to initial codes identified during analysis. In addition, she checked for the accuracy of the representation of participants' voices under each emerging theme throughout the interpretation process, and also provided guidance on ethical decisions at each stage of the research.

Institutional Review Board (IRB). I submitted an application to the University of Montana's Institutional Review Board (IRB) prior to distributing the call for participants. I made revisions to the IRB application based on comments provided by the board. The application and supporting documents such as the participant recruitment email, recruitment flyer, demographic information survey, emergency contact information form, and consent form were all approved by the University of Montana IRB #213-22, and followed the American Counseling Association's Code of Ethics (2014). IRB amendment was requested and approved (Appendix B) to include participant incentives, use of a flyer (appendix E) for participant recruitment as well as utilizing Qualtrics to collect background information and consent from participants. I followed each of the procedures listed in the IRB documents throughout the data collection process and my communication with participants. For instance, participants were informed of their voluntary participation and the fact that they could withdraw from the study at any point without any consequences. I also informed participants about reasons for recording the interviews and data storage procedures. I informed participants about the procedures that might follow in case of crisis situations whereby I would make the decisions collaboratively with them to ensure their safety.

Prolonged Engagement. Lengthy and intensive contact with participants to identify salient constructs representing their knowledge adds credibility to the knowledge (Lincoln & Guba, 2007). To facilitate prolonged engagement, t data collection was conducted in two phases. The first interview was held for approximately one hour with an additional 5 minutes or less follow-up discussion. The longest interview time was 1 hour and 9 minutes while the shortest was 47 minutes with a mean interview time of 55 minutes. Throughout each interview, I noted the facial expressions, vocal tone and nonverbal communications participants were making alongside the verbal description of their experience of the sexual violence encounter and what transpired afterwards. These notes were added in the transcription and included in the quotes under the first- and second-round analyses. I then conducted the initial and focused coding. After exhaustively reviewing the categories, subcategories, properties and dimensions identified during the first-round analysis, I was able to identify the gaps and develop the second-round semi-structured interview questions. During the second-round interview, I informed all the participants that I would reach out to them to share the framework with major findings and would appreciate their feedback and perspectives. They all agreed to be contacted for member checks and expressed their interest in providing their thoughts and suggestions on the findings. The same procedure for transcribing the data and conducting initial and focused coding was used following the second-round interviews.

Once the coding and second-round analysis was complete, participants were contacted for member checking. During this process, I sent the image of the framework of healing from sexual trauma that had emerged based on their experiences of navigating life following sexual violence. This image consisted of the major codes and themes identified by the researcher based on the first and second rounds of data analysis. These continuous interactions with participants provided the opportunity for me to fully engage with the data for an extended period of time.

Member check. Rigor in qualitative study requires the fair representation of the voices and their differences based on their values, co-constructed and portrayed in the study, and can be achieved through member checking (Lincoln & Guba, 2007). Lincoln and Guba (2007) state that member checking ensures that participants' reaction and feedback are included in the reconstruction of knowledge, and is utilized both during the inquiry process by asking for feedback from participants and later, when frameworks are developed during the data analysis process. During both rounds of interviews, I used clarifying questions and paraphrases to check my understanding of participants' process and experience of surviving from sexual trauma as we co-constructed knowledge about the movement within that journey. After the second interviews, I shared my analysis with all the participants to validate the fair and authentic representation of their experience and process of surviving sexual trauma. A rigorous member checking process leads to a strong agreement within the participants that their views and values are fairly represented in the co-construction of knowledge (Lincoln & Guba, 2007).

Triangulation. Creswell and Poth (2018) stated that using multiple methods of data sources enables qualitative researchers to establish credibility of the findings and/or the framework developed based on the data from the field. At the end of the first-round interview, I prompted my participants to share a piece of artwork/photography/spoken word/poetry/song that spoke to their journey of surviving from sexual trauma. The request for a voluntary contribution of artwork was also included in the participant recruitment email and flyer. By the end of the second-round analysis, all of the six participants shared their artwork/photography/spoken word/poetry/song representing their journey. One of the participants shared their art piece immediately after the first-round interview which enabled me to include it during the first-round analysis. As I integrated the art pieces submitted by participants in the analysis, I excerpted parts of the work that spoke to the identified theme except for images and some poems that were included in full to keep their integrity. These pieces of data were used to triangulate the data collected through the interviews, and are included under Appendix J.

Memo. During each interview, I kept a memo of my observations of participants' nonverbals, vocal tone and facial expressions as they described their experience and process of surviving sexual trauma. These memos were used later to inform my reflections on the process of the interview as well as my reactions during the interview. Each memo was part of a discussion with my inquiry auditor and was included in the data analysis to show the participants' unspoken language as they reflected on their experience.

Journaling. The constructivist grounded theory approach requires reflexivity and deep examination of one's values and perspectives (Charmaz & Belgrave, 2018). To improve my reflexivity, I kept a journal focused on the emerging themes as well as my process of flexibility in identifying and deidentifying themes. Appendix K lists some of the major initial conceptual maps that emerged as I constructed the framework of healing from sexual trauma. The journal helped me record and process what was coming up for me as I interacted with the participants, analyzed the data, and interpreted the results. This journal increased my methodological self-consciousness where I recognized and named my worldview, my perspectives regarding sexual violence, and the healing process. My viewpoints were part of the multiple and detailed discussions with my inquiry auditor.

Researcher positionality and reflexivity

According to Charmaz (2017) and Creswell and Poth (2018), qualitative critical inquiry requires researchers to recognize and explicitly state their values, position and power as they interpret the meanings of experiences and processes learned from the participants. Charmaz (2017; 2020) argues that reflexivity, or examining the researcher's identity in relation to the study and developing methodological self-awareness, is key to constructivist grounded theory. Researchers need to practice reflexivity and methodological self-awareness throughout their study as they develop theory based on the findings in the field (Charmaz, 2020). To this end, I here explain my salient identities and positionality as I interacted with the participants.

I am a 36-year-old cis-gendered black woman with a disability. I grew up in a collectivist culture. I was born in a low-income family household that later transitioned into poverty due to familial situations. In my adult life, I was a middle-income earner, and I am familiar with the toll of historical economic disadvantages. Through my experience with acquired disability as an adult, I am recognizing the impacts of ableism on the disability community and noting the environmental barriers enforced by ableist systems and infrastructures. As a teacher and later as a counselor, I listened to countless stories from my friends' and clients' experiences of sexual violence by intimate partners and/or strangers. After moving to the United States, some of my identities that were once in the background became more primary, such as my color and international student status—which comes with temporary legal status and restrictions to some legal rights. On the other hand, my ethnic identity and spirituality moved to the background. Because of these two identities and where I was geographically located, I had held privileges of the dominant group in my country. As I built rapport with my participants in this research, I was aware that I had individuals coming with individualistic cultural values who may have held different privileges and/or underrepresented statuses associated with their positions in their own community. I have seen and heard how economic disadvantages, societal stigma towards sexual trauma survivors, and victim blaming could contribute to the hurt after violence, as well as more victimization of those who are vulnerable. From these stories and experiences, I learned the intrusiveness and pervasiveness of the act of sexual violence.

Moreover, as a person who grew up observing and experiencing different forms of sexual violence, I recognize the ups and downs of processing the experience. Personally, individual therapy, advocacy, reading books, confiding in close friends, and finding connection have been helpful in recognizing the impacts and implementing strategies that helped me engage in my own healing process. I recognize my experience and process of healing, or the meanings I give to these processes may be different from my participants. As a result, I used different means of ensuring trustworthiness of my interaction with participants, the data collected, analyzed, and reported from participants.

Summary of the methodology

In this dissertation, a qualitative research method was employed to collect, analyze, and interpret the data regarding the experience and process of surviving from sexual trauma. Charmaz's constructivist grounded theory was used as a guide to interact with participants and engage in the co-construction of knowledge. Initial sampling, open coding, focused coding, axial coding, and analysis were guided by the principles of constructivist grounded theory. I used Clarke's method of situational mapping to lay out the contexts and relations within the emerging themes during the data analysis process. Member checking, prolonged engagement, inquiry auditing, memo writing, and reflection, reflexivity, and IRB approval were utilized as procedures to establish trustworthiness.

CHAPTER 3: FIRST-ROUND ANALYSIS

For the first-round data analysis, I interviewed six individuals who identified as underrepresented based on their sexual orientation, gender, race, and/or disability status. The interview questions focused on the research question: what is the experience and process of surviving sexual trauma? I used five semi-structured, open-ended questions to guide the interview process, and then asked follow-up questions based on the disclosures the participants made in response to the guiding questions. No specific questions were asked about the type of sexual violence, the perpetrator and/or any of the circumstances involving the event of sexual violence. However, to further explain their experience of surviving from sexual trauma some participants voluntarily disclosed the type of sexual violence they experienced and/or some of the contexts and circumstances around the event. Below is a list of the first-round questions:

1. How would you describe your process of surviving a sexual trauma?
2. Was there a particular moment, or set of events, that really changed the trajectory of your surviving journey? Can you tell me more about that/those?
3. What was something or some things you found especially challenging in your process of healing? What were some things that were especially helpful?
4. Are there moments when your healing has become especially clear to you? What are those?
5. Are there moments when you uncover more work to do, and how do those moments present?

All six interviews were transcribed and uploaded to NVivo version 12. Coding was done word-by-word, line-by-line and incident-by-incident to develop themes that emerged from the experiences of the participants. During the first-round interviews, an initial code book was created incorporating 560 codes. Following the initial coding, focused coding was done to develop major themes that spoke to participants' experience after the sexual violence. During the focused coding process, the initial codes were combined into categories and subcategories, and then dimensions and properties were created to support the categories and subcategories.

Figure 3 shows a conceptual map of themes, subthemes, properties, and dimensions as well as social situations that emerged based on the experience of surviving sexual trauma and its integral contextual- and identity-related factors. Seven major categories (shown as colors; Figure 3) emerged during the first-round interview: **sociocultural contexts, identity exploration and formation, pre-trauma self and relationships, the perpetrator, disclosure, responding to trauma, and moments of relief and empowerment.**

Figure 3

Journey After Sexual Violence and its Contextual Factors

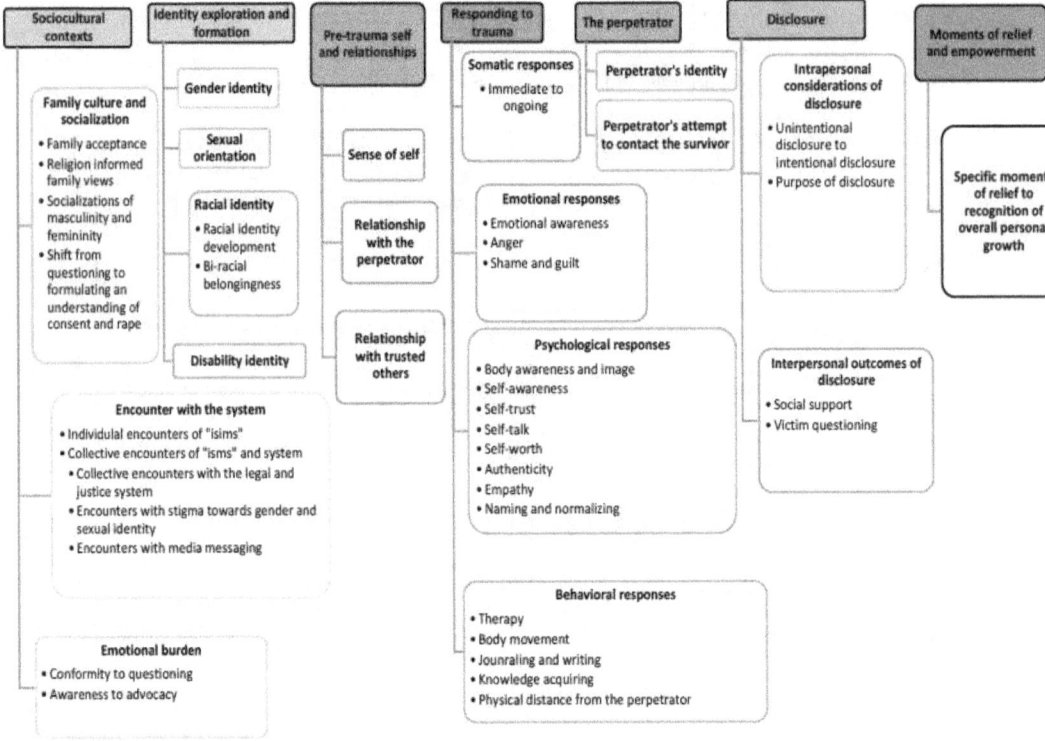

Description of participants

Six individuals who identify as members of an underrepresented group based on their race, sexual orientation, gender identity, and/or disability status were interviewed. Participants' ages ranged from 21 years to 40 years old. The shortest time interval between participation in this study and the sexual violence experience was 7 months, while the longest elapsed time was 17 years. All participants responded "No" to experiencing childhood sexual violence. All participants were asked to choose a pseudonym of their choice and this pseudonym was used during the transcription, coding, and analysis.

Table 2

Demographic Characteristics of Interviewees

Participant Pseudonym	Age	Sexual Orientation	Gender	Race	Disability Status	Time After Event
Nathan	27	Heteroflexible	Male	Asian, Mixed	No	Almost Three Years.
Tim Samson	40	Sexually Oriented Toward the Female Gender	Gender Expansive - Male Presenting	White	No	10 Years
Sophie	37	Queer	Female	White	No	14 Years
Christina	21	Bisexual/Queer	Nonbinary	Hispanic (White)	No	Longest 4 Years Ago, Most Recent 2 Years Ago
Nichole	25	Pansexual	Nonbinary	Filipino American, Pasifika	No	7 Months
River	35	Pansexual	Nonbinary	White	Neurodiverse and mental health problems	17 Years

Nathan is a 27-year-old Asian American mixed-race male who identifies as heteroflexible. He reported no disability at the time of this first-round interview. He shared that he had experienced rape by a white woman almost three years ago. Tim Samson is a 40-year-old male-presenting white individual who identifies as gender expansive. Tim Samson identified his sexual orientation as being oriented towards the female gender. Tim Samson reported multiple incidents of inappropriate sexualized touching for an extended period of time while working in a previous industry, by individuals identifying as both male and female. Tim Samson did not identify as having a disability at the time of the interview and it had been 10 years since the experience of sexual violence. Sophie is a 37-year-old white queer female who reported having experienced sexual violence 14 years ago. She did not report having a disability, although she did disclose being on medication for mental health issues. Christina is a 21-year-old Hispanic white who identifies as bisexual and queer, and non-binary. Christina disclosed using both they and she pronouns. They did not report having a disability and disclosed three incidents in which she experienced sexual violence within the last four years; the most recent of these was two years ago. Nichole is 25 years old, pansexual, Filipino American and Pasifika who identities as nonbinary who uses they/them pronouns. Nichole did not report having a disability and the sexual violence happened seven months prior to the interview. The sixth interviewee, River, is 35 years old, white, and identifies as pansexual and nonbinary. River disclosed a disability status due to diagnosis of neurodivergent disorders and mental health problems. River experienced sexual violence 17 years ago.

Emerging participant experiences

Seven **categories**, written in bold here after, of participant experiences of sexual trauma emerged during the first-round analysis: a) **sociocultural contexts**, b) **identity exploration and formation**, c) **pre-trauma self and relationships**, d) **the perpetrator, disclosure**, e) **responding to trauma and f) moments of relief and empowerment**. *Subcategories,* written in bold and italic here after, and *properties,* italicized here after, were identified to support each **category**. Experiences showing a shift and/or movement in participants' journeys after sexual trauma were included in dimensions that will be underlined hereafter.

The first two categories, **sociocultural contexts** and **identity exploration and formation**, reflect participants' experiences of encountering the situational and contextual factors surrounding their lives before, during and/or after experiencing sexual violence. As a result, not all of the *subcategories* and *properties* or dimensions under **sociocultural contexts** and **identity exploration and formation** are tied to the sexual violence event itself but rather may focus on participants' interaction with their social and cultural contexts as an individual with underrepresented identity(ies). These **sociocultural contexts** and the experience of **identity exploration and formation,** whether related to the sexual violence event or not, are essential factors influencing participants' understanding of the sexual trauma and journey after experiencing sexual violence. Similarly, the third category, **pre-trauma self and relationships,** is focused on participants' understanding of themselves and the relationships they established prior to the sexual violence that shaped their responses following the sexual violence. The other four categories, **responding to trauma, the perpetrator, disclosure, and moments of relief and empowerment,** are specifically related to participants' experiences during and/or following the sexual violence they encountered.

Here I will first describe the overarching social and cultural situations that emerged and were categorized as **sociocultural contexts** as participants explored their identities and navigated the journey of sexual trauma. These social and cultural factors that intersected with and were foundational to participants' experience of navigating the journey were coded as parts of the situational analysis.

Sociocultural contexts

The **sociocultural contexts** category refers to the norms and cultures of upbringing and participants' understanding of sexual violence and trauma. This category also includes the participants' experience of navigating social and cultural contexts as both a survivor of sexual violence and an underrepresented group member. Participants discussed the significant roles of family norms, knowledge of consent, and being accepted within their social context in recognizing a transgression as sexual violence. As individuals engaged in the process of self-exploration and identity formation, the messages they received within their immediate relationships and larger family contexts played a significant role in their experience with exploring and forming their identities as well as responding to trauma.

Participants discussed the challenges they experienced due to systemic policies and underlying cultural norms that limit their authentic presence. They learned acceptable identities and behaviors through the family norms and the messages they received when they were young. Larger contexts such as societal and media portrayals of identities have also impacted their authenticity and self-worth. Participants' journeys of identity formation and experiences of sexual violence were also impacted by national social justice movements. Participants discussed the constant fear they feel for their safety and the hypervigilance as they navigate the cultural expectation in relation to their religion, legal status, and race intertwined with their experience of sexual violence. The participants' experiences also reflected three *subcategories: a) family culture and socialization, b) encounters with systems,* and *c) emotional burden*. Below is the detailed description of participants' experience with the sociocultural contexts.

Family culture and socialization. The *subcategory* of *family culture and socialization* refers to family norms and cultures that shape the actions and perspectives of participants as they explore their identities and make everyday decisions. Cultures surrounding religion, place of origin, and family norms centered around care and acceptance influenced how participants viewed themselves. Four participants discussed their perceptions of their family and religious culture while growing up:

> **Tim Samson**: If I was to be approved of ... accepted if not a problem, and I'd be approved if I was exceptional.

> **Christina:** I come from a Catholic family, a Mexican Catholic family, so Roman Catholic, and who, at times, had some very traditional views...
>
> **River:** they were-they [parents] were hippies in the 70s and my mom was like "yeah I never wore a bra" and she's like "and then "I wonder why men would whistle at me."
>
> **Nichole:** I grew up in a fundamentalist Christian setting that saw bodies as being for certain thing um kind of praised certain types and didn't praise other types...um maybe that has to do with like my immigrant upbringing too like grandma's like always commenting on the grandkid's appearances and stuff.

These participants' childhood experiences have influenced personal decision-making and development of a sense of self as survivors navigating the challenges of adulthood. These family norms not only influenced the participants' sense of self, but later informed a variety of decisions participants made and shaped the process of exploring identities and determining expectations about themselves. The perceived judgement and approval from adults in the participants' early life shaped the image participants created for themselves and their body. As Nichole indicated above, the understanding of their body was shaped by how adults perceived their body and comments they received when they were young. Participants' understanding of sexuality and sexual behavior was also shaped by how these behaviors were modeled to them by their parents.

Specifically, two participants shared the struggles of meeting the expectations of their family culture and norms as they explored and came to terms with their own identities and decisions:

> **Tim Samson:** So, a lot of the choices I made growing up were like be exceptional, be exceptional, be exceptional, be Aragorn from the fucking *Lord of the Rings*.
>
> **Christina:** Yeah, absolutely. So, when it came to gender and sexual identity, I come from a Catholic family ...and that definitely made it hard for me to come to terms with myself. Just who I was or who I am.

Moreover, Christina shared the family norm and culture around expression and management of emotions. This *family culture and socialization* had posed a challenge for Christina as she was intending to disclose her experience with sexual violence to her family:

> **Christina:** And sometimes it's difficult to get emotions out of my parents, as I mean, my mom comes from, well, she's from Mexico. So, she has that, like Latin background, and my dad comes from basically an emotionally unavailable family that doesn't talk about their feelings. It is so, like going into that [disclosing sexual violence] ... I didn't really know how they were going to react, and I think that honestly made my healing process a little bit harder.

The *subcategory* of *family culture and socialization* consisted of three *properties: a) family acceptance, b) religion informed family views c) socializations of masculinity and femininity* and a <u>dimension</u> of shift <u>from questioning to formulating an understanding of consent and rape.</u>

Family acceptance. This *property* of *family acceptance,* under *subcategory* of *family culture and socialization,* refers to participants' perceptions of being accepted and acknowledged by their family in both the presence and absence of disclosure of their identities. These participants' perceived parental acceptance and approval shaped their experience of identity exploration mainly regarding gender identity and sexual orientation. The pressure to fit in with the culturally and religiously accepted identities created a challenge to explore and/or authentically present their identities to the world. By contrast, survivors who perceived their parents to be accepting of their identities had been able to come out to their parents and reported a smooth conversation:

> **River:** and my mom even knew [my sexual orientation] from a young age, and I thought it was funny [smiling] and when I told my dad he was ...I told him I had a boyfriend... he was like he was "damn you mean you're not gay?" like "I'm gonna have to worry about you getting pregnant?"

Religion informed family views. The second *property* under the *subcategory* of *family culture and socialization* was *religion informed family views*. This *property* represents participants' perception of the role of religion in shaping their family's views and their conceptualization of underrepresented identities. The socially learned stigma against individuals who identify as gay, and perceptions of body image, posed a challenge in coming to terms with sexual and gender identity. Specifically, religion informed perspectives enforced by parents, and contributed to the narratives survivors created about themselves, thus contributing to the challenges faced in forming an identity and image of their body. Two participants provided details of the impact of learned behaviors at an early age:

> **Christina:** And I had learned about that [being gay] before, like when I was still in elementary school, like or middle school, my dance teacher had come out... her [participant's mom] exact word, ...sounding like "that's not our family." ...which means 'that's not me,' which means 'I can't be gay.'
>
> **Christina:** and then going through that like mental turmoil of like, 'well, I am gay. So, what do I do now?'
>
> **Nichole:** I... I isolated myself from situations where people would be able to see me using my body basically and that came too with, I mean I grew up in a fundamentalist Christian setting that um saw bodies as being for certain thing um kind of praised certain types and didn't praise other types.

Socializations of masculinity and femininity. The *family culture and socialization* messages can also be tailored towards gender identities mainly focused on the understanding of masculinity and femininity. This participant's experience is represented under the *property of socializations of masculinity and femininity*. Participants talked about the impact of socially learned perspectives in shaping their understanding of consent and safety as well as the tendency to assume responsibility for being a victim, even after experiencing violence.

> **Tim Samson:** I think there was something about the me being a man in that situation [sexual violence] or male presenting I was like 'oh, that doesn't happen! this is just...'

> I do not identify as man...I had those cultural experiences. I mean it was like [chuckle] 'boys being boys!'
>
> **Sophie:** I think females because we tend to manage trauma and trauma disorders by convincing ourselves that we could have done something differently.

These *family culture and socializations* specific to *socializations of masculinity and femininity* have also shaped how survivors named and understood their sexual violence. Participants discussed the difference in their pre and post sexual violence understanding of sexual trauma. They also shared the shift they needed to make in how they defined sexual violence and trauma as they created meaning from their experience. This shift in knowledge and understanding of consent is captured under the dimension of shift <u>from questioning to formulating an understanding of consent and rape.</u>

Shift from questioning to formulating an understanding of consent and rape. This <u>dimension</u> describes the shift in participants' knowledge and understating of consent and circumstances surrounding rape following sexual violence and/or after being able to recognize and name a sexual encounter as violence. One participant, for instance, shared that the early messages on safety and consent have affected their effort to keep themselves safe from the perpetrator:

> **River:** I remember when I was a kid ... my mom would explain to me "don't walk down a dark alley at night or something [will] grab you and rape you" and like you know so that's like the visual of it that I had. It was always like a violent attack from a stranger...obviously that is not the case...

Two participants, one identifying as male and another as male presenting, talked about their perceived invincibility to sexual violence before their own sexual violence. This perspective led to denial and had prolonged their experience of naming what happened to them and led to repeated questioning of the validity of their sexual violence experience:

> **Tim Samson:** It [sexual assault] really was …. something that I thought was culturally normal.
>
> **Nathan:** because I think that … I think that as a man and as someone who identifies as a man um…there is this particular culture that says that when a woman likes you or wants to do something sexual with you it's a good thing… and it ultimately validates your existence as someone who is masculine.

As a result, due to the *family culture and socialization* surrounding male sexuality, Tim Samson and Nathan questioned the validity of their perception of their sexual violence by either thinking the sexual violence is "normal" or "desired." For Nathan, the experience of questioning was expressed through doubts about participants' perceptions and memory, and physiological reactions to the transgression:

> **Nathan:** '…maybe I'm leaving out details' or 'maybe my memory is faulty' or… because you know that there's … I've taken so many different psychology classes that have talked about how memory is faulty and that was something that I was always really concerned like 'maybe I'm just misremembering.'

In addition to questioning the validity of their memory, participants also attempted to give a meaning to the unwanted sexual attention by interpreting it as an indication of their desirability and acceptance:

> **Nathan:** I remember thinking 'maybe it [sexual violence] was… maybe it was a good thing maybe…maybe it proves that I'm desirable.'
>
> **Tim Samson:** I definitely… I don't look the way that I looked when I was getting all of this attention [the sexual violence]. And that became such an identifier for me like "[Tim Samson] is one of the best [professionals] in [metropolitan city]. Everybody wants to fuck him" and like that was such an identity.

This questioning the validity of experiences with sexual violence was not specific to male presenting or male participants. Another participant talked about the questioning of the validation of their sexual violence experience after others question the intention of the disclosure of sexual trauma:

> **River:** Yeah, it's like 'am I overreacting? Am I…am I just jumping?'…

As a result, participants needed to make a shift in their shift <u>from questioning to formulating an understanding of consent and rape</u> and sexual trauma after experiencing sexual violence themselves. They needed to learn new concepts on consent around sexual encounters to be able to trust their perception of their reality. For Nathan, it was important to remember the "context" of sexual violence to be able to name the sexual encounter as traumatic:

> **Nathan:** But then I remembered the context of it, and I remembered how it wasn't a mutual exchange...

For River, to shift <u>from questioning to formulating an understanding of consent and rape,</u> it was important to have external validation and evidence to name and normalize the sexual encounters as a sexual violence experience. This validation came from local and national social justice movements that helped create a new understanding of consent and rape:

> **River:** when the #MeToo movement happened, it started reframing everything and I was like 'oh, that's why that [sexual violence] like messed with me. That's why I felt that way towards that [sexual violence event] situation' because it was like 'oh, I'm not just being dramatic' like 'this was actually a thing that happened.'

Participants shared that knowledge and understanding surrounding consent has been helpful to objectively evaluate the sexual violence event and determining that they were wronged. Related to the shift in understanding of consent and trauma, Nichole and Nathan talked about the importance of educating oneself about the meaning and parameters of consent, and the trauma responses as essential components to help them shift the blame from self to the perpetrator:

> **Nathan:** ...but then I remembered the context of it, and I remembered how it wasn't a mutual exchange... it was something that happened, and I froze and tensed up and it happened so fast.... at least it felt like it happened so fast.

> **Nichole:** ... that like that's... it [rape] wasn't... it wasn't rape ...it was ...I didn't say anything so it's my fault, you know, like I can ...can imagine not having been educated about sexual assault would have affected me.

Other participants needed those closest to them or professionals they were working with to name and validate the event as sexual violence and assault, and as traumatic, before beginning to shift their understanding of what happened to them. Tim Samson discussed the help of his therapist in naming and acknowledging the sexual violence he experienced:

> **Tim Samson:** ...so, we were just, in our work [therapy], I started talking about those instances [sexual violence] in those events. She was just like "I am going to stop you for a second here [gesture of blocking] what you're describing is a) assault and b) the way you are describing it, it sounds like it traumatized you" and that hit me like a freight train.

The shift <u>from questioning to formulating an understanding of consent and rape</u> was helpful since, in some circumstances, participants needed to justify the lack of consent as they disclosed their experience to others. One participant shared their experience of justifying the presence and absence of consent to their loved ones as:

> **River:** when I talked to my mom about it [rape] she was like "see I wouldn't have considered that rape" and I was like 'yeah, but there was no consent...but I never said yes. I never wanted it. I was scared to say no' and she was like "oh" she's like "I mean obviously it is but..." she's like "I never would have [considered the event as rape]."

As depicted in the above participants' voices, the *family culture and socialization* provide a framework for how participants understood their experience of sexual violence. Participant's perception of being accepted by their family have positivity contributed to their identity development. The *family culture and socialization*s were influenced by *religion informed family views* that the participants' family held, and the messages and norms created in the family in accordance with these religious views. Participants also discussed the role of *socializations of masculinity and femininity* that shaped their understanding as they explore and formulate their perceptions on gender identity and expression. The *family culture and socialization*s also shaped participants' shift <u>from questioning to formulating an understanding of consent and rape</u> that needed to positively change before starting the process of healing from sexual trauma. These *family culture and socialization*s are often shaped by larger socializing constructs that both the participants and their families are exposed to including religion and generational understanding of consent and rape. As a result, participants consistently encounter the larger system as they explore and form their identities and respond to the sexual trauma.

Encounters with the system. The second *subcategory* under the sociocultural contexts was *encounter with the system*. This *subcategory* explains survivors' experience with the larger norms and systems that impacted their experience of identity formation and informed their decision whether or not to interact with the justice system after experiencing sexual violence. Specifically, under this *subcategory*, experiences of "isms" and past encounters with the police and judicial system were discussed by participants. Some of these experiences were individualized while others represented more collective experiences as survivors of sexual violence or as members of an underrepresented group. In addition, some participants discussed the intersection of their identities with surviving sexual violence. To capture these intersections and experiences, two *properties* were created under the *subcategory* of *encounter with the system*: *individual experiences of 'isms"* and *collective experiences of "isms" and the system.*

Individual experiences of "isms". This *property* is defined by participants' disclosure of being targeted because of their identities by the perpetrator and/or people around them. Targeted negative actions of others towards the participants' identities sometimes intersected with their experience of sexual violence. For instance, Nathan, who identifies as an Asian American mixed-race male, specifically discussed the details of the pre- and post-sexual violence conversations with the perpetrator. He discussed his belief that his racial identity was targeted and objectified, and this left him to wonder, especially during his early stage of trauma recovery, whether his race caused the sexual violence:

> **Nathan:** I remember her [perpetrator] commenting on that I was ethnic that I was Asian and that made me attractive in a sense and I don't know if that was one of the reasons that it happened or transpired but I do remember …I do remember thinking 'that's weird!'

Nathan also recalled that his race was used to degrade him after the sexual encounter. This personal experience of insult directed at his racial identity and body size resulted in Nathan's later consistent questioning of his racial identity and self-worth:

> **Nathan:** I remember she [the perpetrator] touched my cheek and she said, "why are you shaking?" and I [do] not say anything "you don't like me?" I didn't say anything still and she got off of me and she scowled at me, and she said "you are just a short Asian guy anyway" [silence] …. [tears & long silence] …I guess to be told that you're short and just an Asian guy, it's kind of like, so that means that I am easily disposable or something?... and I do not know its [deep breath] …[silence]

The aftermath of *individual encounters of "isms"* creates persistent self-consciousness and a sense of shame. In Nathan's experience, for example, the race-based insult created consistent and prolonged shame about his body:

> **Nathan:** and I am now constantly aware that I'm short and I have often felt very ashamed that I'm short… and I've been ashamed that I'm short because I'm Asian and it all tied to this one moment because before that I never really thought about how short I was.

For other participants, the **encounter with the system** occurred collectively as they witness others experience these "isms" and/or other negative experiences. These *collective encounters of the system* had a significant impact on their decisions and actions following their experience of sexual violence.

Collective experiences of "isms" and the system. This *property* refers to participants' collective experience with individuals in the legal system and/or navigating the judicial system with others. There are three *sub-properties* under the *property* of *collective experiences of "isms" and the system:* a) collective encounters with the legal and justice system, b) encounters with stigma towards gender and sexual identity, and encounters with media messaging.

Regarding the collective encounters with the legal and justice system, participants talked about their past personal experiences as well as the experience of witnessing others' struggles with the legal and judicial system. None of the participants I interviewed talked about seeking justice through the legal system. Two participants detailed their firm decision to *not* involve the police or legal entities responsible for reporting because of their past experience with the legal system or those involved with it. Nichole and River, both of whom identify as pansexual and nonbinary, provided details of past encounters with the legal system and attempts to report sexual violence that impacted their decisions not to involve the police or any part of the legal system after experiencing sexual violence:

> **Nichole:** the first time I walked through something like this [reporting sexual violence] with friends, she had been sexually assaulted by someone that we knew…and we were all in school at the time, so we filed it as a Title IX…it just became too challenging for it to sort of like remain anonymous um… it just became gossip too.
>
> **River:** in New Orleans in 2006, there was a few of us sitting outside this bar waiting for a show and three cop cars showed up, and …we were wearing dirty T-shirts and stuff, we were just traveling and they told us all [to]line up on the wall, and like searched all our pockets and the girl next to me, the cop was like reaching his hands like as far as he could in the pockets and she was like trying not to cry and he was like "what's wrong? Did your daddy touch you too much? Or did he not touch you enough?" and at that point I just wanted to like, obviously you don't punch cops, but in my head [I wanted to punch the cop]... And then he's got to me and firmly grabbed my breast, and then like search my back pockets. I had nothing.

For River, experiencing sexual violence in 2006 and witnessing sexualized verbal/emotional abuse by the police informed their later decision to avoid any encounters with the legal system.

> River: 'ok, I guess that's just how they [the cops] treat women'... that was kind of just like 'ok, I'm gonna do everything in my power to stay away from them [cops] now'

In a similar vein, Nichole chose to manage the pain of sharing physical space with the perpetrator for a period of time after the sexual violence rather than involving the law. This decision was informed by existing systemic oppression against people of color:

> Nichole: I'm obviously brown and then other ways obviously queer too... like whoever whatever like white cowboy was going to be the one handling the case ...basically, I just didn't want to be the recipient of any more evidence of the world is the way it is. [laughter]

In addition, Nichole's past experience with reporting a friend's sexual violence informed their decision to not go through the "tiring" process of seeking justice despite having the knowledge of how to report and where to go to seek justice:

> Nichole: there were ways for me to have someone put control over that situation [sharing a house with the perpetrator after the rape], I just like could not even fathom, you know, like trying to get the law involved or like police or things like ...it just like...felt like so tiring.

> Nichole: any sort of like formal [laughter] process...um... that had gone poorly for my friends in the past and so for such a limited amount of time it's like 'this is just gonna be fine', but I did feel like pretty intensely unsafe for that month.

Another *sub-property* under the *property* of *collective experiences of "isms" and the system* was encounters with stigma towards gender and sexual identity. Participants discussed their *collective experiences of "isms" and the system* in terms of the early exposures to stigma targeted towards participants' sexual and gender identity. One participant disclosed their early encounter with stigma against sexual diversity and their effort to keep themselves safe and protected:

> River: I feel like everyone [in grade school] was like so just weirded out [by River's sexual and gender identity] it's like "oh there was a weird person that exists at our school" and then like my friend Megan started dating a girl, and it was like, and then suddenly like the school was like "wait, there's more" ... I was never physically

attacked because of that [sexual identity] or anything but like, I still felt like I needed to have my guard up.

This cultural stigma towards sexual identities was also reflected in how the law and policies are formulated by ignoring the need to keep sexual underrepresented individuals safe from sexual violence. One participant discussed the discouraging policies that negatively impacted the effort to report sexual violence as a sexual minority:

> **Sophie:** but since we so often in the US don't think that women having sex counts as sex, then I imagine that sexual violence in any gay relationship is likely underreported probably the same with men too, I mean especially in [western United States], doesn't count as rape or statutory rape if they are the same gender.

As a result, underrepresented individuals find themselves in a situation where they need to advocate for their human rights to be respected, just like those in dominant groups. However, these advocacy efforts were met by "pushbacks" from members of the dominant culture. As an example of this pushback, Nichole shared a petition written against gender- and sexuality-affirming policy changes at a previous college they attended:

> **Nichole:** the institution that I was attending and working for before this, Presbyterian school, just there's been a bunch of drama this week because there was a petition written, people think by either one of the board members or someone close to the board, that is just like deeply homophobic.

During the interview, Nichole seemed greatly confused about the reasons for this pushback to gender- and sexuality-affirming policies; they shared the survivor's emotional burden that underrepresented students carry having been compelled to advocate for their own rights to be respected:

> **Nichole:** this is wild [petition against queer rights] and so ... then there was a counter policy ... written by mostly students I believe, like queer students ...and it's like 'this is ridiculous.'

These consistent, mostly negative, *encounters with the system* influenced participants' decisions not to seek justice, despite the negative consequences of sexual violence. As a result, participants as individual survivors of sexual violence carried the burden of coping with the trauma without legal justice.

The *collective experiences of "isms" and the system* were also discussed by participants in the ways media misrepresents behaviors associated sexually underrepresented groups. This phenomenon was represented under the third *sub-property* of *collective experiences of "isms" and the system* as encounters with media messaging. Sophie, who now identifies as queer and used the term bisexual in the past, discussed the trauma caused by the misunderstanding of bisexual sexual behaviors by those in the entertainment industry that leads to misrepresentation of bisexual sexual behaviors:

> **Sophie:** …as someone who is bisexual or whatever attracted to more than one gender…represented in media including in queer media of being um…promiscuous which of course has its own stigma.

These messages of "promiscuous sexual behaviors" involving those who identify as bisexual, based on Sophie's experience, were also repeated in personal experiences of romantic relationships. Sophie shared the impact this misunderstanding and misrepresentation of sexual behavior had on her self-worth and understanding despite these portrayals not representing her values:

> **Sophie:** so yeah, "whenever it's someone who's bisexual it means you can't trust them" which that I get to internalize. There is this constant extra shaming of don't even trust yourself in sexual situations.

> **Sophie:** I happen to be a very monogamous person probably more about attachment issues than philosophy [chuckle] but…

The internalizing of these messages, according to Sophie, negatively impacts her ability to authentically represent her sexual identity and behaviors during romantic encounters:

> **Sophie:** so that kind of the sexual references about you are untrustworthy…you're inherently untrustworthy when it comes to sexuality is a piece that is intertwined with my own comfort and being sexual in any given situation.

These messages of mistrust towards the bisexual identity are also repeated in the personal experiences and attempts to connect with others. The voices of mistrust towards those who identify as bisexual come from both heterosexual men and lesbian women:

> **Sophie:** and you know, yeah, there is, yeah, there is a lot of resentment there and I'd say I felt it from... I can't think of a lesbian woman who I'm friends with that hasn't expressed their level of distrust ...um... and straight males those are the ones who are most threatened. Straight males are like "well, what if a female could do something that I can't" you know "what if I'm not enough" is where it comes from.

This questioning towards bisexual trustworthiness had affected Sophie's self-worth. She described the internal experience of feeling unvalued and unwanted by others including those closest in her social circle:

> **Sophie:** definitely some of the kind of lowest moments I've had outside of just the joys of depression but just like independent episodes have been when people who are close to me have unknowingly [chuckle] said such devaluing things about what someone like me could do based on being bisexual and just feeling in that moment like a ...um...yeah... like unwanted by... unwanted by society.

In general, participants described their *encounters with the system* as unpleasant and as deterring them from making positive steps towards healing from sexual trauma. They disclosed how both *individual experiences of 'isms"* and *collective experiences of "isms" and the system* have negatively impacted their journey. Because these *encounters with the system* are embedded within the participants' **sociocultural contexts** influencing their **identity exploration and formation** as well as understanding of sexual trauma, as members of underrepresented culture, they carried the *emotional burden* of having to advocate on behalf of others who may be victims of the system.

Emotional burden. The third *subcategory* under the **sociocultural contexts** is *emotional burden*. *Emotional burden* refers to the experience of navigating the nuances of norms established by both the dominant and underrepresented cultures, and the necessities and felt responsibilities to question and advocate. Participants' experiences ranged from a general sense of "feeling activated" to realizing the survival nature of advocacy. They also discussed the pressure they felt to express and inform others of their identities as they established and maintained their sense of belongingness. This included recognizing their own privileges and identities that are impacted by the "isms" within their **sociocultural contexts** as they carry the *emotional burden* of advocating. The experience of *emotional burden* was described by two dimensions indicative of participants' experience of making shifts in thoughts and actions: conforming to questioning and awareness to advocacy.

Conforming to questioning. The dimension of conforming to questioning refers to the experience of recognizing personal values and privileges and moving to questioning the validity and responsiveness of the existing cultural norms and systems. Some participants shared that the shift from conforming to the dominant cultural perspectives towards questioning them came after experiencing sexual violence. Several participants, however, shared that their experience of moving to a new community and entering a new cultural norm of relative acceptance of diversity facilitated their process of questioning. These new cultural norm encounters provided the opportunity for participants to move from conforming to the dominant perspective and the negative consequences, to the process of questioning and advocating:

> **Nathan**: I transferred my credits to this school and it was my first semester… and I was getting used to the political climate …because it's very different than where I lived before and [place of origin] is far more conservative than [current city] is and the political climate here is more liberal. There are people who are more open to all these different things like the more open to feminine struggles and, you know, the environment and racism and like over in [place of origin] people are really conservative.
>
> **Nichole:** and I was like 'ok, great I've had all this built up like anxiety and insecurity around sports and physical activity. No one here knows me. I'm gonna go and find

something, and if I don't find it now, I'm never going to' so my first couple months here I visited every single yoga studio in town.

For some participants, the transition from <u>conforming to questioning</u> was impacted by the nuances of moving to a new city and starting a new career, each of which may be accompanied by a lack of understanding in the new circumstances of the personal boundaries and understanding of consent. One survivor detailed the confusion around setting boundaries as they joined a new workplace culture and the assumptions they made about sexual boundaries:

> **Tim Samson:** so like getting married and then moving to [metropolitan city] its where all this [sexual violence] happened was eye opening because it was basically the first, I started to build this career [in a previous profession], and like the very first show that I was cast in was one where I was experiencing some tough harassment and 'oh, well, big city, new career, this is how you do it!'

The realization that the professional norm does not have to involve nonconsensual sexual advances has helped Tim Samson to recognize his experience as sexual trauma:

> **Tim Samson:** coz I came in [previous profession] as an adult, so it was not like… I did not grow up in that culture and be like 'oh this is how people are' and yeah …and it turns out it's not. It doesn't have to be, or even if it is how they are, it was…it impacted me pretty directly.

The process of identifying areas where participants have questions regarding their identities as well as the norm of sexually inappropriate behaviors, provided the opportunity to strengthen their personal awareness.

Awareness to advocacy. This <u>dimension</u> refers to participants' experience of gaining knowledge regarding their identity, values, and sexual trauma to move towards advocating both for themselves and others. Participants described the relationship between personal awareness of their values and identities as underrepresented members, and their advocacy efforts. One participant talked about the consistent state of questioning their personal decisions: should they advocate, or if they chose not to advocate would their silence be considered as being complicit with the oppressive norms and cultural practices?

> **Sophie:** I think a lot of times I am just in general activated because I can either be part… contribute to the aggression or I can just say what happens to be true for me [oppression]…

Participants also discussed the added *emotional burden* of advocating for one's identity as a member of underrepresented groups. The *emotional burden* of advocacy comes from having to constantly speak out and perform to validate their existence and promote acceptance within their sociocultural context:

> **Sophie:** .um…I think the queerness of being perpetually just like invalidated from straight and gay people makes it feel like I need to be…um….an activist just to be um…[silence – trying to find words] just to exist… like I would …I would expect a male someone who's trans male to talk more about their masculinity [than] someone who was born male.

> **Nichole:** then there was a counter policy written that's like written by mostly students I believe …like queer students… it's like 'this is ridiculous.'

The transition from personal awareness to advocacy was also facilitated by the insights gained after experiencing sexual violence. Nathan discussed in great detail how his experience with sexual violence contributed to the *emotional burden* as he disclosed his experience and, at the same time, encouraged him to advocate for those who might be subjected to sexualized stigma and violence:

> **Nathan:** however, there have been times that I've pressed myself to talk about it [sexual violence] because I do feel like it is important to acknowledge that these types of things happen to men.

> **Nathan:** it's really made me more empathetic. I care a lot about people's feelings ever since this [sexual violence] happened…and I'm far more likely to tell men if they're acting a certain way like "you shouldn't do that" … far more likely to care about others' feelings.

Overall, participants discussed the **sociocultural contexts** that influence both the experience of **identity exploration and formation** as well as their journey after sexual trauma. The *family culture and socialization,* the first *subcategory* under the **sociocultural contexts**, shaped participants' perspectives on acceptable identities and behaviors. Moreover, based on their *family culture and socialization* participants formed a <u>shift from questioning to formulating an understanding of consent</u> that needed to shift so they could start creating meaning from the sexual trauma. In the second *subcategory*, participants also shared the negative *encounters with systems* that sometimes are *individual experiences of 'isms"* and other times *collective experiences of "isms" and the system.* These *encounters with systems* have impacted the decisions of reporting sexual violence and negatively impacted their experience after sexual violence. In the third *subcategory, emotional burden,* participants discussed their shift from <u>conforming to questioning</u> of social norms and then from creating <u>awareness to advocating</u> for themselves and others. These **sociocultural contexts** have provided a foundation for an understanding of their journey after sexual trauma as well as exploring who they are and forming an identity that is congruent with what feels right internally and externally.

Identity exploration and formation

The second **category, identity exploration and formation,** emerged based on participants' experience of navigating the journey of sexual violence. Similar to the **category** of **sociocultural contexts**, not all *subcategories* of **identity exploration and formation** are directly connected with the participants' experience with sexual violence; rather, they capture the experience of meaning making in relation to one or multiple participants' identities before and after the sexual violence encounter. Participants discussed their experience of exploring their sexual, race, gender, and disability identities and the intersection of these identities with their **sociocultural contexts** as well as the experience of sexual violence. This category is connected to participants' experience of navigating the journey after sexual trauma and efforts to become more authentic about who they are and how they present themselves to the world. The **category** of **identity exploration and formation** has four *subcategories*: a) *gender identity, b) sexual orientation, c) disability recognition,* and d) *racial identity.* Each of these subcategories is elaborated below based on the experiences of participants.

Gender identity. When discussing *gender identity,* participants addressed the circumstances that enabled them to explore these and to express their gender. For some participants, the initial encounter with the terms and labels of gender identity was met with surprise and curiosity. Two participants talked about the consistent curiosity they had as they encountered materials, labels, and discussions around gender before forming their current gender identity:

> **Tim Samson:** I've always been interested in gender studies. I took the gender studies program.... why am I .... I'm always ever the only straight white guy at every single one of my classes...'why, why do I do this? Why do I care?'

> **Christina:** ...then, being like, 'Whoa! Whoa! Gender...gender! What's that? Oh, oh, we're going to be switching that around' like figuring out...

While Christina and Tim Samson shared the process of naming and exploring their *gender identities,* another participant discussed the pressure of gendered expectations and binary gender expressions. For Nathan, educating himself and realizing that congruence within gender identity and expression is associated with his happiness have helped him to push back on potential stereotypes about expressions of masculinity:

> **Nathan:** for example, my hair is green, and two years ago, I would have never done my hair a funky color like this but after reading these books and thinking 'I should just be whoever I wanna be because people who are who they are [are] happier.' I had this

confidence to just kind of 'I'm gonna dye my hair. I am gonna wear colors like pink... I'm gonna pull off these styles and I don't think that affects my masculinity at all.'

This self-assurance and authentic expression of his masculinity has helped Nathan to be happier.

Other participants also discussed their self-reflection about *gender identity* and moments of realization regarding where they fall on the gender spectrum. For instance, Tim Samson disclosed the power of self-reflection on gender identity and the relief experienced during the moments of congruence:

> **Tim Samson:** ...and like I was out on a hike, and I was sitting by myself, and I realized, like out here I don't feel male, like I feel ...me and I am not defined by the society's construct of what it means to have a penis. and that really was.... God, it feels good!

Following this realization of nonconformity to the gender binary norms of the society, participants were able to name and create their personal meaning of *gender identity*. Exposure to labels and names for *gender identities* helped with the process of coming to terms with their gender identity:

> **River:** ...nonbinary popped up...[I] was like 'that's me'...
>
> **Tim Samson:** And then I hear of the term gender expansive... 'Oh... wow [surprise and eagerness] 'what this?... 'Tell me more about this, this feels like me.'

While Tim Samson was able to attend classes to educate himself on gender and sexuality and had the opportunity for a personal space to reflect on what feels congruent rather than conforming to gender binary stereotypes, another participant shared that exposure to a supportive social environment has facilitated their process. Nichole stated that being around those who were able to authentically express their gender identity has created an opportunity to start their process of nonconformity with society's expectations of gender identity and expression:

> Nichole: when I was separate from this highly heteronormative [culture] realizing that like 'oh, I also want to talk about this [gender identity]' and I'm realizing like 'this is a safe place for me to just' like 'maybe they pronoun would be good once in a while for me.'

Participants also shared that the process of understanding gender as fluid rather than binary has been an ongoing and slower journey. Both Christina and Tim Samson discussed their ongoing process of coming to terms with the fluidness of their gender:

> Christina: ...I do identify as like a nonbinary woman... I still feel very girly, but there are definitely like days that I'm not girly. So, figuring that out. And then with that, and like becoming comfortable in both my masculinity and in my femininity.

> Tim Samson: Tell me more about this [gender expansive], this feels like me. I don't.... I don't feel like a man. I don't feel like I am. I don't walk through the world thinking 'man'. I walked to the world thinking feeling like me, and like some days that's very flowy.

Participants shared that time, space, and support from others where they feel accepted has helped to authentically engage in the process of **identity exploration and formation**. Two participants disclosed that the support of a trusted social network enabled them to engage in the process of *gender identity* exploration:

> Nichole: [I] found myself next in a place where like I could add on to that different understanding of gender and sexuality. It was like universe skydiving whatever is going on in this world that had given me different contexts slowly come into an understanding of myself...how these intersectional layers [come together] and also a community that supported me walking through those layers too.

> Tim Samson: I will feel myself go to that [femininity] place and to some level it is comfortable. When I am like that around women it is not sexualized and I can be just like ...oh...soft and societally feminine in a way that feels really authentic and like grounded, and I can feel kinship with the feminine.

As Nichole and Tim Samson stated, acceptance by others facilitated their experience of *gender identity* exploration. At the same time, the expression of gender around those who are perceived to be unsafe for those who identify as gender underrepresented can be problematic.

Christina, who is a Hispanic white and uses she/they pronouns, shared that advocating for her pronouns has been especially hard when around those who identify as men:

> **Christina:** Mmhmm. Yeah, and honestly, I...it's harder to, at least for me, it's been harder to like express that I use they/them pronouns, or like I prefer they/them pronouns over she/her pronouns to people who identify as men.

Moreover, as Hispanic white and bilingual, Christina's experience attempting to use preferred pronouns may have been complicated by language and grammatical incorrectness when proper pronouns are used. Therefore, Christina found a way to address her personal preference of pronouns and ways to fit to the dominant culture:

> **Christina**: ...and as a queer non-binary... I still say, woman, because then I should use ...like she they pronounce mostly she, because Spanish it's so much easier and not grammatically incorrect to just use feminine pronouns.

In general, the experience of *gender identity* exploration was facilitated by the curiosity and readiness of participants to explore their gender and move away from conforming to the gender binary culture and norms of society. Moreover, the process of *gender identity* exploration was supported by participants' perceived acceptance by those around them upon disclosing their identity to trusted others.

Sexual orientation. *Sexual orientation was* identified as the second *subcategory* under **identity exploration and formation**. Participants discussed the process of exploring their *sexual orientation* as they also encounter the **sociocultural contexts** that, at times, facilitate and, other times, hinder the process of forming their sexual identity. Two participants shared that their experience of exploring *sexual orientation* was intertwined with their understanding of gender:

> **Christina**: ...kind of realizing, like gender is kind of dumb, and as long as a person intrigues me, and I enjoy spending time with them, it shouldn't matter.

> **Nichole:** down here I'm with these a bunch of like gay poets [laughter] and I was like I think I am like you, you know, and [I] found myself next in a place where like I could add on to that different understanding of gender and sexuality.

Similar to the experience of gender identity exploration, participants also discussed the importance of social support as they explore their sexual identity and disclose their romantic interests. Christina talked about the support from her sister and friends that provided an opportunity to normalize her *sexual orientation* and express herself congruently:

> **Christina:** my sister, has been the most accepting and supportive person ever like... uhm...didn't even question it when I was like 'yeah, a girl'... she like "that's cool. what's her name?" I was expecting so many more questions. She's like "no dude, that's fine." So, her, my sister, and my best friend have like...they've been the main supporting people for me.

> **Christina:** So, my friends have been very supportive in that they're just like "Woo, go! Whoa, yeah, is this a part? Who? non-binary, guy, girl, who are we talking to today?" and I'm like this person, they're like, "okay, cool! what are their pronouns?" and I'm like "this," and they're like "Sweet, okay, continue on with your stories." So, like having them be so supportive and like open to me figuring all of this out has been so helpful.

Similar to the ongoing process of exploring *gender identity*, participants also shared the continuous nature of exploring *sexual orientation*. Two participants related the ongoing nature of exploration of *sexual orientation* and identity:

> **Christina:** and then going through that process again of like 'okay, maybe I do like guys. What does that mean for me? Do I still like girls? Well, yes, do I like guys now, I guess. If a non-binary person is around, would I be fine with that? Well, yeah. So like, then I still like the gay like gay label. I don't know why, but that's, that's the label that I still like... it's still kind of like in my brain. I'm like "No, I don't want to like men, but at the same time I do," so it's, that's still process...we're working on it...

> **Sophie:** I...I used to say bisexual but now I don't see gender as that binary, but I don't so whatever.

One participant, however, talked about the clarity they had around their *sexual orientation* but were not able to name it because of the lack of proper language to express *sexual orientation*. River described the experience of "knowing" sexual preference and identity long before they were able to name and label their identity:

> **River:** um...I knew I was queer from a very young age.

Based on the participants' experience of exploring *sexual orientation*, they were able to recognize that acceptance by significant others and the **sociocultural context** allowed opportunities to continue with **identity exploration and formation**. Similar to *gender identity* and expression, *authenticity* in *sexual orientation* has positively facilitated the journey after sexual violence.

Racial identity. Participants of color also talked about their experience with racial identity development; therefore, a third *subcategory* of *racial identity* was created under **identity exploration and formation** to represent their experience. Both Nichole and Nathan discussed their experience of navigating making meaning of their racial identity as they interact with their **sociocultural context**. Both participants shared their realization of the meaning others give towards their color of skin. Nathan, who identifies as Asian American and mixed, discussed the early image of his racial identity as mostly formulated based on the messages from those around him. Nichole, who identifies as Filipino American/Pacifica, shared the realization of being different based on their color of skin shaped by the experience of immigrating to the United States:

> **Nathan:** you know, I never really liked being Asian as a kid because when I was seven or eight, I was told to go back to my country you know I was born in this country and [tears].

> **Nathan:** I've often felt like my eyes been tied directly to my race.

> **Nichole:** I knew vaguely that like I'm brown [laughter] that means something different in the continent [America] [laughter].

There were two *properties* identified under the *subcategory* of *racial identity*: *racial identity development* and *bi-racial belongingness*.

Racial identity development. One of the *properties* of *racial identity* was the experience of the *racial identity development* through the discussion facilitated by local and national social justice movements. These movements created a space where participants were able to focus on their *racial identity development*. For Nichole, further exploration of *racial identity* was facilitated by the social justice movements against anti-race violence and police brutality in the United States. They shared the experience as:

> **Nichole:** at this last school it felt like my primary self-journey was about race and sort of coming to an understanding of what my ethnic heritage means to me and how to talk about it with other people. This was like the summer of George Floyd and Brianna Taylor and so I was like you know able to participate in that conversation and felt called to it in a way that I hadn't been previously.

Bi-racial belongingness. The second *property* under the *racial identity subcategory* was *bi-racial belongingness*. Depending on the intersections of racial identities, participants needed to navigate the sense of belongingness to each culture. Nathan explained the struggle as a mixed-race individual trying to fit into two independent racial identities: White and Asian:

> **Nathan:** I know what it's like to have like an Asian grandma who... I know what it is like to eat rice with every meal, you know, ...I also know what it is like to have... have never been considered white by white people, that makes sense [chuckles] I know... I also know what it's like to be considered solely white by the Asian side of my family is ...is kind of horror.

To further complicate matters, the race-based insult and objectification that happened to Nathan during the sexual violence incident has negatively affected his views towards being an Asian American. Nathan recalls his perpetrator's statement of "you are just a short Asian guy anyway" and its long-term negative impact on him:

> **Nathan:** I've been ashamed that I'm short because I'm Asian and it all tied to this one moment because before that I never really thought about how short I was.

This led Nathan to consistently compare his body, especially his height, with others around him and amplified the thought that he is different and does not belong. Nathan detailed his tendency to look at other people's height to normalize his body size, which he believes is tied to his racial identity:

> **Nathan:** know that my dad my dad is he he's 5'3... and he's Chinese and Filipino and when you go over to the Philippines like the average height is like [my dad's].

> **Nathan:** one thing that I am constantly...[chuckling] ... people in [western United States] are so tall like there are so many people here in [western United States] are just really, really tall ...my brother lives in NYC and you go there people are my eye [level] people are shorter ...some people are tall but like there's a wide range here in [western United States] I feel like everyone's really tall and I just feel really small all the time .. and ...I never felt small before that incident [sexual violence] I never even I thought it was an issue.

Nathan's and Nichole's experiences expose how personal encounters with racism and witnessing others experience racism contributed to their difficulty in developing a secure sense of belongingness. As a result, for these two participants, their *racial identity* has been a salient factor as they give a meaning to their sexual violence experience.

Disability identity. *Disability identity* is the fourth *subcategory* identified under the **category** of **identity exploration and formation**. Only one participant identified as having a disability. This participant, who identifies as having a disability due to Autism/ADHD/Panic Attacks, discussed the signs of autism they were able to recognize early in life with some of these signs reflected in their social interactions:

> **River:** I [did not] know I'm also autistic so it's like I feel like that might come with like ... I don't have the same like social boundaries and stuff a neurotypical people have...so I never, even though it was like the early 2000s, I never was like felt weird about it.

> River: um...I [silence – thinking] and I have read that like autistic people you know have a lot of them have trouble lying and are like very like what most people call brutally honest I've been called that so many times in my life and I don't always mean to be brutal it's just to me it's just honesty it's just like fact.

However, the lack of early diagnosis contributed to the confusion and lack of naming their experience. River stated that having a diagnosis that helped them label their symptoms has been validating and self-assuring:

> River: yeah and I also and I always like because like I figured out I was autistic before I got diagnosed and my therapist was like when she actually like you know confirmed it and like did all the tests and stuff and she was like "well how do you feel about that?" and I almost like started laughing I was like "I feel validated [high pitch to emphasize being validated] yeah like I was like and I feel pretty clever of figuring it out [laughter].

After the experience of sexual violence, River believed that having a diagnosis for autism has helped them to process traumatic experiences and create meaning:

> River: everything made sense in different ways, and I was like 'well!' and like after that I found it easier to process more traumatic things that had happened to me because I had a different like framework in my brain.

River shared the long wait to get diagnosed with Autism and reflected on the importance of early diagnosis to help people with disabilities to have a framework for navigating life. The disability identity development for River has focused on recognizing the signs and being able to name them.

In the experience of **identity exploration and formation**, participants discussed the role of the **sociocultural contexts** in either facilitating or becoming a barrier to their identity development. They disclosed the importance of social support and authenticity as they explored and formed their identities. Participants also discussed the barriers such as racism and cultural expectations that hindered their process of forming a sense of belongingness. As participants discussed their experiences following sexual violence, they also reflected on the personal work of forming their identities and the values they held before experiencing this trauma. Although participants did not specifically discuss the intersections of their multiple underrepresented identities during the first-round interview, most of the participants shared more than one underrepresented identity.

Pre-trauma self and relationships

The third **category** that represented participants' experiences was the **pre-trauma self and relationships**. The **pre-trauma self and relationships** is defined by participants' sense of self and their understanding of their relationship with others before they experienced the sexual violence. Participants discussed the relationship between their understanding of themselves, principles of boundary setting, and their relationship with the perpetrator as factors intertwined with their journey after experiencing sexual violence. They also discussed the importance of having formed trusted relationships that facilitated their effort to ask for help once the violence occurred. There are three *subcategories* under the **category** of **pre-trauma self and relationships**: *sense of self, relationship with the perpetrator* and *relationship with trusted others*. I will discuss each of these subcategories below.

Sense of Self. This first *subcategory* is explained by participants' disclosure of the understanding of identities, values, and awareness of themselves as they interacted with the rest of the world prior to the sexual violence experience. One participant discussed the role of self-awareness and formulation of values as a protective factor to minimize the length and severity of negative trauma responses:

> **Nichole:** and I think it... it ...it the event [sexual violence] occurred after a really formative period in my young adulthood where I had developed a pretty strong sense of self and like a...a sort of confidence that I didn't have when I was younger. I also had a really high view [of myself].

For another participant who was in the early stage of developing their sense of self when they experienced sexual violence, the process of recognizing one's values needed to happen before working on traumatic experiences:

> **Tim Samson:** and thinking to myself like, there's no reason that I can't be like Aragorn...there's nothing standing in my way like "I'm a good, gentle person. I've really artistic sensibilities. I also love the outdoors and feel strong and... I had this realization...just like idealized mythological character... 'What's holding anybody, let alone me back, back from trying to live as this?' ...I think, it was a stupid thought [chuckles], because I both held myself to certain standards, and also, like ignored certain qualities about myself that like....um...I need to work on that.

For Tim Samson, being at the early stage of developing a sense of self was associated with accepting unwanted, inappropriate and nonconsensual sexual advances as part of a culture and not advocating for oneself.

> **Tim Samson:** ...moving to a place where I was approved of in a very specific way, but it was just the way I looked ...I didn't have to be a unicorn. I just had to be in a room...

For Nathan, on the other hand, the self-reflection on the pre-trauma self and relationships involved reassessing the values he wanted to hold onto as he integrated sexual trauma into part of his life journey:

> **Nathan:** I guess....um...[silence] you know I.... before this [sexual violence] happened, I would say .... that I... I'm gonna be honest ...I'm gonna be real with you before... my before.... my... before I experienced sexual assault, I feel as if I had objectified women more and I had thought of women to a lesser extent or more as like object.

All of these statements that participants disclosed about the values and images of themselves they held prior to their experience of sexual violence, both for themselves and others around them, impacted the way they processed their traumatic experience. Participants also shared the relationships they had with the perpetrator prior to the experience of sexual violence.

Relationship with the perpetrator. The *relationship with the perpetrator* is the second *subcategory* under the **pre-trauma self and relationships**. Four participants shared that the perpetrator was known to them, and that they have formed a trusted relationship with the perpetrator prior to the sexual violence encounter. Of these participants, some shared that they had formed a trusted relationship with the aggressor:

Nichole: my aggressor was a housemate.

Nathan: had just started being friends with. She [the perpetrator] invited me to hang out with her... I was like 'I'm not doing anything. why not... it is something friends do.' I didn't think that it [hang out] was weird.

River: it was someone I went to high school with, someone I had known since middle school I was like; you know, we had the same circle of friends and felt like, he was...I mean he was very manipulative even like as a friend.

Tim Samson: this one [person in power] in particular...he was very attracted to me.

Tim Samson: a good friend from college, and I knew him before he was out [came out as gay] ...we went to a club, and so much fun... the end of the night has come...touched [me] in ways that feel really inappropriate and it felt really boundary crossing...And my friend was like "haha..come on" like he was like really mad at me for not wanting to go along with it ... he took advantage of me.

These participant disclosures show that the existing relationship with their perpetrator contributed to participants' trust that the perpetrator would not wrong them. In Tim Samson's case, the positionality of the perpetrator also played a part in how he perceived the sexual violence.

Relationship with trusted others. Pre-trauma self and relationships was also associated with the formation of *relationships with trusted others* before the sexual violence occurred; these relationships served as protective factors once participants experienced the sexual violence. Participants talked about the sense of protection and safety they gained from relationships that were established prior to the sexual violence. These trusted relationships facilitated the process of disclosure and trauma recovery:

> Nichole: yeah… let's see…um… the first person I called was someone from my program actually a classmate of mine who is older and who is a mom ..um…and with whom I had already shared a lot of my um a lot of my story <click> [stress on the prior strong relationship that was trusted]
>
> Nichole: I did also reach out to those people who I was who are no longer in proximity with me but who know even more of the story and have seen me and even more circumstances that have been difficult and have also seen me um change over time.
>
> Christina: …and she's [a friend] been with me through, 2 out of the 3 events [sexual violence] …has supported me.

These trusted relationships that were established and maintained by participants before their experiences with sexual violence have helped them to ask for help and gain support. As mentioned above, these social supports are indicated as positive experiences for participants as they responded to sexual trauma.

This **pre-trauma self and relationships category** provides an important insight about the role of participants' positive *sense of self*, as it helps to reassure them during the process of naming and normalizing their response to the sexual violence. Participants shared that they have formulated a relationship with the perpetrator, both formal and informal, that contributed to their trust to their perpetrator prior to the sexual violence encounter.

Responding to trauma

The fourth **category** that emerged from participants' experiences was **responding to trauma**. This **category** refers to both the negative somatic and emotional reactions following the experience of sexual violence as well as their psychological and behavioral experiences as participants make meaning of the transgression they experienced. Most components of **responding to trauma** were reported as individualized and internal experiences as participants navigated trauma and encountered both triggers and facilitators during their recovery journey. As participants reflected on how they responded to the sexual trauma, they disclosed its cyclical nature in which triggers can elicit raw somatic and emotional responses whereas positive experiences lead to relief:

> **Christina:** Yes...ummm, two moments [that changed the trajectory of the trauma recovery, and the first one was the first time that the person [perpetrator], like the first person, they reached out to me again, and that, like, almost sent me back to square one like. It was not a great.
>
> **Sophie:** um...I definitely struggled with the embarrassment and then self-shame which then fuels the insecurity whenever I do have this panic sobbing shaking response you know so um...yeah... I think that perpetuating a sense of lack of control over my own body by having these traumatic reactions...

As Christina and Sophie indicated, despite having the skills to manage trauma responses, triggers can lead to a refreshed negative trauma reaction. Some of these triggers can be related to the meaning participants gave to the negative trauma responses.

The experience of **responding to trauma** was explained as both inward and outward responses, with four *subcategories*: *somatic responses, emotional responses, psychological responses,* and *behavioral responses.* Due to the complexity and cyclical nature of participants' journey after sexual trauma, I specifically created another image for **responding to trauma** to show the connection and cyclical nature of *subcategories, properties* and dimensions (Figure 4). All of the *subcategories, properties* and dimensions depicted in Figure 4 show the same *subcategories, properties,* and dimensions represented in the conceptual map (Figure 3) but with emerging processes.

Figure 4

The Experience of Responding to Trauma

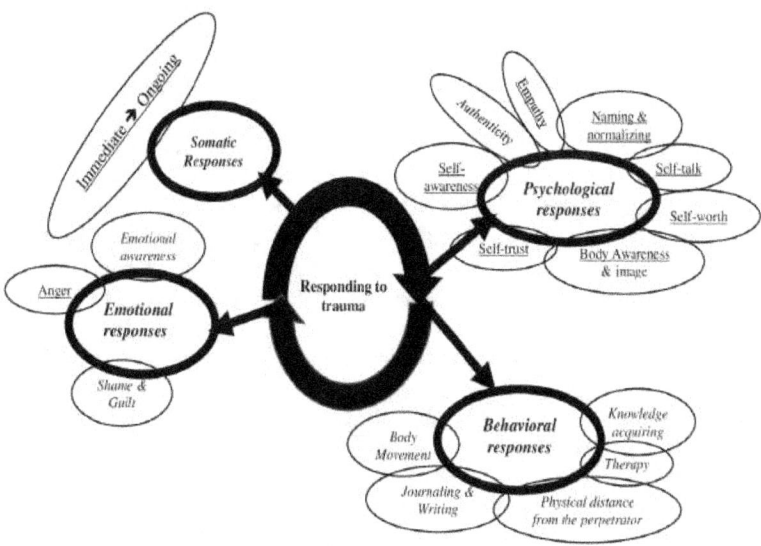

Below is a detailed description of participants' experiences as they responded to the traumatic experience related to sexual violence. The description will start with *somatic responses* and then *emotional responses* because participants shared the occasional overlap of these two. I then continue with *psychological responses* followed by the last *subcategory*, *behavioral responses*.

Somatic responses. The *subcategory* of *somatic responses* is explained by the experience of physiological responses following the sexual violence incident. Participants discussed *somatic responses* both during and immediately after the sexual violence. They also shared the ongoing nature of these *somatic responses* following sexual violence. To capture the ongoing nature of these somatic experiences, I created the dimension of immediate to ongoing.

Immediate to ongoing. This dimension refers to participants' report of physiological reactions during and after the sexual violence experience. One participant disclosed that their ability to recognize the *somatic responses* to sexual violence was connected to their developed body awareness prior to the sexual violence. This body awareness has contributed to Nichol's attunement to their body signals during the sexual violence encounter:

> **Nichole:** so, in the incident [sexual violence] like I was already getting the signals like 'this is not right'...I already knew how my body communicated about ...I don't really have other ways to talk about it ...other than like a like a total memory for like how it...how it sounds when my body [signals me nonconsensual sex].

Two other participants talked about their understanding of how their body responded during the sexual encounter as "freeze." Nathan added the perception of time during a trauma response:

> **Christina:** um...I froze. Everyone says it's like fight or flight. It's fight or flight, or freeze, and I've froze.

> **Nathan:** ...then I froze up. I don't really remember all that happened, but it felt like it happened really fast and then simultaneously felt like it happened really slow...I was shaking.

Another participant shared the high intensity of the somatic reaction following the sexual violence. This participant did not specify the details of the *somatic response* rather gave a general description of the experience as:

> **Nichole:** ...obviously the emotions and like the physical experience was intense...

Participants also discussed the ongoing nature of these *somatic responses* to sexual violence. Some participants disclosed their encounters with generalized triggering events leading to a full panic reaction while others discussed specific triggers associated with their inability to self-regulate. One participant discussed these ongoing unpredictable *somatic responses* that sometimes occur during consensual sexual encounters:

> **Sophie:** ...something that happened with lots of people since my sexual trauma which is just this full on like just a panic attack like shaking, dissociation, hyperventilation all that kind of stuff.

Another participant shared that the ongoing *somatic responses* are triggered when he finds himself in a setting where he, as a male sexual trauma survivor, feels unheard and unseen due to the greater focus on women sexual trauma survivors. As a result, he often "dissociates" to cope despite the urge to speak up and advocate on behalf of those whose experience is not shared and being discussed:

> **Nathan**: …it's isolating… it kind of feels like… moments like that [moments of feeling unseen and heard] happen it kinda feels like everything around me becomes fuzzy and numb, and I just try to silence everything out, and I try not to hear it… and I try to just stay inside my thoughts even though I know my thoughts consistently tell me that it's wrong, and that I should be saying something.

These ongoing *somatic responses* are also shown in gastrointestinal responses to trauma. One participant talked about a chronic somatic response to trauma:

> **Tim Samson**: …of course, you have somatic symptoms, you know, and you know, digestive stuff like, anyway.

In general, participants shared that their body awareness has helped them to recognize *somatic response* to trauma. Moreover, they disclosed their *somatic response* as the sexual violence is happening as well as immediately afterwards. Ongoing *somatic responses* are associated with triggers participants experience following the sexual violence.

Emotional responses. The second *subcategory* in the **category** of **responding to trauma** was *emotional responses*. Participants discussed experiencing ongoing emotional reactions to the sexual violence. They shared feeling anger, hurt, shame, fear, and guilt at different times during or after the sexual trauma. Most participants were able to name anger and shame and guilt as the common *emotional responses* to their traumatic experience. As a result, two *properties* and one dimension were created under the *subcategory* of *emotional responses: emotional awareness, shame and guilt,* and anger.

Emotional awareness. This *property* is defined by participants' ability to recognize, invite and manage their emotions related to the sexual violence experience as well as emotional reactions to daily stressors. Two participants discussed the lack of experience and skills, due to past learned behaviors, to intentionally allow themselves to feel emotions; this may have added complexity to the processing of their sexual trauma and disclosing their experience to others:

> **Nathan:** I was in an argument with my partner and then like as we were arguing I just kind of like broke down and it just came out [disclosed sexual violence].

River, on the other hand, shared a learned coping mechanism related to emotions:

> **River:** yeah, well, my family is big on using humor as a coping mechanism which a lot of people look at me weird. I'm like 'hey if it works it works.'

As a result, participants needed to learn to allow themselves to feel negative emotions despite their limited intentionality to feel emotions before the sexual violence. For some participants, this *emotional awareness* came with their ability to be intentional about feeling their emotions and this contributed positively to their journey following sexual violence:

> **Nichole:** yeah, and that's like science or something, right, I read somewhere that like chemically emotion last a certain amount of time and like any prolonging of that is me …[laughter] at least I think that's how it works. If it's not how it works, I don't want someone to tell me.

> **Christina:** I'll let myself have like a… it's full night like after dinner time. I make sure that I eat first, so that I do eat, and I'm not like too emotional to not eat if that makes sense. So, dinner first, and then, after dinner, all the emotions can come on out.

> **Christina:** it's. It's weird to feel emotions like actually in your body. And I'm not always the best about it. So, I still make sure to do it every once in a while, but like actually take time out of my day or out of my week and be like 'okay, we are feeling emotions today. How are we feeling?' And then let that might go how it goes.

Participants' ability to recognize and allow themselves to feel emotions not only related to the sexual violence but also other challenges of everyday life has contributed to their *emotional awareness*. Among these emotions, *shame and guilt* and <u>anger</u> have been commonly identified by participants.

Shame and guilt. Another *property* under *emotional responses* is *shame and guilt* felt frequently by participants. Participants disclosed several sources of shame about the sexual trauma. Shame can be related to self-blame for not protecting oneself from the perpetrator or can be related to how participants responded and are responding to sexual violence. One participant shared that shame was expressed through covering their body to protect others from potentially noticing the participant was sexually violated:

> **Nichole:** after that I was like T-shirt, long leggings, keep on... keep my sweater on or something. I just felt like, so uncomfortable being seen as if like someone could tell that I'd been assaulted.

Another participant described the consistent shame as an emotional reaction whenever she has panic reactions to sexual encounters following sexual violence:

> **Sophie:** ...then I went through this whole shame thing about ... 'why do this?' it's super unsexy to start crying and these moments [physiological trauma response during sex] ... and 'I'm very sick.'

A third participant disclosed the shame he feels as he reassesses and reflects on the values he had and may have used to relate to others; a fourth participant shared the shame about conflicted emotions while the ongoing sexual violence was occurring:

> **Tim Samson:** it [sexual violence] felt kind of good that is part of the shame like... the anger [towards] myself. I can let myself be like molested like as an adult... like... what the fuck [Tim Samson] you know better like but you also liked it but you hated it at the same time."

Some of the *shame and guilt* was related to the views participants held prior to their experience with sexual violence:

> **Nathan:** yes, feeling guilty about how you might have been or who you might have been or views you may have held.

Participants also talked about the ongoing nature of these *emotional responses* to sexual violence, some triggered by the memory of how the violence occurred to them and/or thinking about the circumstances surrounding the sexual violence:

> **Nathan:** um...like images or replay [the sexual violence] in my head and start to feel really anxious and emotional.

> **Tim Samson:** And also, you also get the shame...shame every day like while you go to the gym like "why am I going to the gym? what are you doing to yourself? ... just do it for health, do it for health, do it for health... don't do it for vanity." Anytime I have vanity, I am like "why do you care?"

One participant disclosed that part of the shame following the sexual violence was tied to his race due to the perpetrator's insults about his body and race:

> **Nathan:** so, I've often felt like my eyes been tied directly to my race and I am now constantly aware that I'm short and I have often felt very ashamed that I'm short and I've been ashamed that I'm short because I'm Asian and it all tied to this one moment [sexual violence] because before that I never really thought about how short I was.

As a result, the *emotional response* of *shame and guilt* was related to a variety of issues including internalization of insult by the perpetrator, trigger responses, and self-blame following a sexual violence.

Anger. This dimension was described by participants as one of the common and ongoing *emotional responses* due to the meaning they give to the sexual violence. Two participants discussed that the anger they feel about their experience with sexual violence. In Tim Samson's experience anger is expressed through withdrawal while Christina shared the shift from self-blame to anger as she started to create a meaning to her experience with sexual trauma:

> **Tim Samson:** and it [anger] would show up in ways where I'd be like...I would just need to be alone, or I want to take a nap, or like anything I could do to avoid feeling that type of arousal...

> **Christina:** after [sexual violence encounter] like... self-blame, I turn to anger...

Another participant shared that the anger they feel is targeted towards the perpetrator and at times triggers thoughts of confronting their perpetrator. The participant did not share their anticipated goal for confronting the perpetrator, and the anticipated unresponsiveness of the perpetrator has limited them from attempting contact:

> **River:** yeah, I do have times where like I am still pissed off about it [rape] and wish that I like [reach out to the perpetrator] ... but it's like 'what would I gain from messaging him?' Nothing! ... it's like he would just like... laugh and be like "you're full of crap" and then like probably just made me feel worse but I realized like I don't need to confront him...like he doesn't...he doesn't deserve my time.

Four participants disclosed the anger and resentment they felt and continued to feel towards those who share similar identities with the perpetrator or towards the dominant system they consider to have contributed to their sexual abuse. This ongoing anger is exacerbated by the perceived unresponsiveness of the dominant culture to the participants' desire to see some level of equality and equity for all:

> **Nathan:** um...I started to become increasingly resentful towards women and that was because I started to see that women at the school don't think particularly highly of men at least in my experience I'm not gonna generalize [to] anyone because I think it's wrong to generalize.
>
> **Sophie:** so, in terms of it being like a healing journey I think my journey might just be continuing to say what pisses me off and that might even just be maintenance and not even just part of the journey, but you know.
>
> **Nichole:** Oh yeah. Um (pause) I have this just, like maybe it's well founded for other reasons, and I don't know exactly if it's a useful emotional experience yet, but I just like have this rage against this white...het (heterosexual)...men. (laughs).
>
> **Tim Samson:** I have a lot of anger toward the patriarchy because a lot of the reason that this happened to me is because people were so shoved into this corner... so I can feel real like big rage about like...come on like... this whole system is so fucked.
>
> **Nathan:** I remember really, really angry all the time I come home from class after hearing a classmate of mine speak out or talk about something and it almost came to a point of like I was just angry and really hateful, but I think that that anger and hate came from a place of hurt and a place of like I wish I was seen.

Some of the hurt, anger, shame, and fear shifted into righteous anger, as indicated in participants' experience using anger as a protective tool to assert and maintain personal boundaries and to advocate for themselves and others who are hurting. Righteous anger was also discussed by participants as an ongoing emotional reaction to the experience of sexual violence:

> **Nichole:** I was able to be upset for myself as my own friend as well like [assuring voice] I am like trying the language that… the language of support and care that my old friends would use toward me.

> **Nichole:** so like when someone touches me in a way that I don't like it sure there's anger that gets me to say like "I don't like that" [laughter] that's the moment where the anger is helpful and after that… it needs to turn into something softer because this is the person that cares about me and doesn't understand [where] the reaction is coming from and so … like realizing that we're not going to be able to have a productive conversation about that [anger and assertion] interaction unless I let go of the anger…

Two participants disclosed the anger they felt during in-person encounters with the perpetrator following the sexual violence. They also shared their emotional challenges when they found themselves having to share a physical space with the perpetrator:

> **Nichole:** yeah, I have seen him [perpetrator] a couple of times. It wasn't…not as intense as I anticipated it being but maybe because I have this sort of like shield of protective anger [laughter] whenever… whenever that[seeing the perpetrator] has happened …um yeah, I just tried to tell myself like "I'm for you to be in this space and I guess you are too but like over there" [gestures a physical distance] [laughter].

> **River:** which just made me roll my eyes, and I totally saw him [perpetrator], we totally ignored each other and but like the whole time that I was supposed to be, like, enjoying this show of one of my favorite bands I was thinking about that bastard that was walking around…

Participants also shared their ongoing work to manage *anger* and direct righteous anger towards those who may deserve it instead of generalizing the experience. One participant discussed the internal question of where and when to use anger towards the perpetrator's identity and all who share similar identities. Another participant questioned the usefulness of ongoing anger for their self-maintenance:

> **Nichole:** I don't know where to put that anger (Laughs). But that does feel like work that needs to be done because I do have like dear friends who are not that person...about whom I still make assumptions based on my exper(iences)- past experiences with white men, right? So, it's just, um (pauses) yeah maybe that's the end of the thought; I know that there's work to do there, yeah.
>
> **Christina:** and then, realizing that anger is just not useful in like...it's not like useful use of my energy, it's not productive. I don't need to be angry with the people around me if I've healed. It shouldn't be affecting me so why be angry?

Some participants discussed how these emotional responses, mainly anger and shame about the sexual violence, contributed to their *psychological responses*. This *subcategory* under **responding to trauma** was sometimes tied to the *somatic responses* to sexual violence:

> **Christina:** kind of moving from self-blame or moving away from self-blame. But then noticing in myself, going towards anger, and then again going back to the book and being like, okay? Well, what does he say about anger? And then shifting into like, finally being at peace, and what I felt was like actually healed from that.
>
> **Sophie:** um...I definitely struggled with the embarrassment and then self-shame which then fuels the insecurity whenever I do have this panic sobbing shaking response.

As indicated in the participants' statements, the *emotional response* of anger is ongoing and can be accompanied by shame and embarrassment. Anger can be directed towards the perpetrator, those who share similar identities with the perpetrator, and/or general injustices and underrepresentation participants experience as sexual trauma survivors.

In sum, participants discussed an increased level of *emotional awareness* that has been helpful in their journey following the sexual violence. Participants shared the ongoing anger and *shame and guilt* they felt after having experienced sexual violence. Some of these *emotional responses,* like righteous anger, have been beneficial for setting and maintaining boundaries. The participants also disclosed the relationship between these *emotional responses* and the *psychological responses,* as one can feed on the other.

Psychological responses. The third *subcategory* under **responding to trauma** is *psychological responses*. Participants disclosed the meaning they created about who they are and the values they want to adhere to as they navigate the journey of life after sexual trauma. Some of these internal conversations and understandings of self are the result of and/or associated with the negative *somatic responses* and *emotional responses* the participants had following the sexual violence. Positive *psychological responses* to trauma such as positive self-talk can help participants to experience a moment(s) of relief and self-empowerment. The subcategory of *psychological responses* has dimensions of body awareness and image, self-worth, self-trust, self-awareness, empathy, self-talk and naming and normalizing, and a *property* of *authenticity*.

Body awareness and image. This dimension refers to the experience of an elevated level of body consciousness and participants' view of their body after encountering sexual violence. Some of this hyperawareness and sensitivity to body consciousness was discussed in terms of body size needed for keeping themselves safe. Two participants shared their safety concerns related to body size. Specifically, Sophie shared the risks of safety for a "female" body from male perpetrators by explaining that men's biological ability to "penetrate" creates more risk to a "female" body compared to the risks potentially posed by a female perpetrator:

> **Christina:** Oh, yeah. yeah, I'm cautious with everyone, but especially with men. mostly because of the size difference… I am small, and I think I'm strong, but they're more likely stronger.
>
> **Sophie:** yeah I think there is that piece like a…um… it's gonna be harder for a female body to force itself into a male body so you can get as close as possible without actually penetrating… so I think there's that component that on top of men often

having more muscle mass and you know and that piece and women being submissive and all of those things one thing that's interesting

Having a positive <u>body awareness and image</u> was described as a useful tool to strengthen positive conversation with oneself. However, this level of positive <u>body awareness and image</u> came only after continuous work on self-image and work to become content with one's body. Nichole recalled the positive shift that happened in their body image prior to experiencing sexual trauma.

> **Nichole:** …grew up…um just like very, very deep self-loathing and like body image things and was bullied for my weight and all this stuff that caused me to just not respect myself really ..um…and one product of that is that I didn't participate in physical activities around others because I just kind of like sequestered myself…I isolated myself from situations where people would be able to see me using my body basically…I remember, you know, just like days I would just like stand in the mirror and like self-degrade [nervous laughter] as I'm getting dressed… um and I think …I think it was… I think it was because I wasn't spending quality time with myself and didn't really understand the reasons my body was the way it was. It was more just like an obstacle to what …what I wanted to be the kind of person I wanted to be around it was like an obstacle to like every single like romantic partnership that I had pursued in the past… [because of yoga] I grew into a new spiritual understanding of my body too and like [I] was excited about …about just my body for what it is [giggling] and a way that I had not experienced with physical activity at any other point in my life, seriously like it wasn't until the age of 24 that I found that [laughter], yeah it's crazy

This positive body awareness and image has contributed to a smoother journey after Nichole's experience of sexual violence. Nichole further discussed the relationship they have with their body as a "friendship" that provides consistent support as needed:

> **Nichole:** .um…yeah and in the paying attention like finding out and like just like learning and becoming interested in my body's rhythms and like pay attention to how it communicates to me…um it's just it's the same as having a friend or a partner [laughter] except it's like right here all the time.

Nichole also reflected how their perception of the sexual violence and the experience following that would have been so much different if they have not been able to build a positive body image before the trauma:

> **Nichole:** um... I also um over the past two or three years ..um...have just really developed a love for my own body and like feeling free in it and expressive and understanding it better but before it was an evil thing to be. I just like... I understand it...I thought it was a bad thing and like I didn't... I hadn't learned to value it yet and so if that [sexual violence] happened to me, it would have been like 'whatever ...it's...my body is bad anyway.'

Other participants disclosed the ongoing nature of struggles with body image even after implementing personally preferred interventions to address this struggle. Tim Samson, for instance, shared the challenges he faced trying to make peace with others who considered him attractive, since his physique had been central to the sexual violence he experienced:

> **Tim Samson:** Yeah. So, like the struggle is probably, the biggest challenges have been identity body issues about the image...but I feel like...the comment somebody made ...I shaved. I just had a mustache. This person just like turns out they like mustaches, and they're like "God...you are so handsome." And I was like [holding breath and sign of shock] really felt bad. So yeah. even though I want to look handsome...somebody mentioned something today about how good I looked. And I had the same feelings coming rushing back like 'I know this is a very innocuous compliment...'Thank you. I'm flattered.' I didn't say any of this, and I didn't want burden them like. But also, I was like 'fuck it. I do not want to be defined that way again' but really kind of like pigeon holed. 'Okay? Well, now I gotta show up and be attractive for you.' Yeah, so that that's been hard.

And, despite the dedicated personal work to address the impact of body image on regular and consistent negative awareness of body, he still worries about how others would perceive him:

> **Tim Samson:** and that vanity part is something that like I'm... it really .... it's frustrating like, because I'm... I know that it's not who I feel inside it's...I'm still trying to like... I have this idea in my mind, like 'if I go to [metropolitan city] like and I see any of those people, they are going to have this judgment towards me'.... '[they] be like "what happened to [Tim Samson]? He used to be..."

This ongoing body awareness and image led participants to attempt to change their appearance. Nathan, a 27-year-old Asian American, disclosed his efforts to alter his height so he can appear taller like those around him. This consistent negative body image triggers shame about racial identity:

> **Nathan:** I wear lifts in my boots now [touching and indicating his boots]. I am only like 5'6 ~5'7 and I feel very ashamed that I'm short all the time…

For some, like Tim Samson, this consistent self-consciousness and the negative body awareness and image was not perceived to have impacted their sexual behavior and sexual encounters with trusted others. Tim Samson shared his tentative perception that his body image and identity struggles have not impacted his current sex life:

> **Tim Samson:** It [body image] hasn't....as far as I can tell.... had a huge impact on my sexual relationship with my wife.

However, Sophie shared impact of the negative body awareness and image in relation to her current engagement in sex. Specifically for Sophie, sexual encounters are filled with consistent hyper-awareness of body rather than being able to enjoy or be fully present in this intimate interaction:

> **Sophie:** …I've also… I've never had orgasm in my whole life and that can …I know that's more normal than you know people say it is anyway but I… in sexual experiences very much not present not …I wouldn't say dissociative as more as like de-realized where I'm just kind of like I'm more so thinking about the other person and how I'm presenting than I am about, you know, anything that's happening certainly to my body.

In sum, participants shared their experience with their *body awareness and image* both in relation to the sexual violence as well as in their process of identity formation. Positive body awareness and image facilitated personal growth and facilitated their recovery from sexual trauma.

Self-worth. The second dimension under the *subcategory* of *psychological responses* is *self-worth*. Self-worth refers to participants' belief that they are good enough and worthy of receiving love both from themselves and others around them. Self-worth, both positive and negative, was experienced by participants as they attempted to integrate sexual violence into their understanding of themselves. For instance, Sophie disclosed that her experience of "derealization" during sexual encounters was associated with the intersection of the sexual violence with her sexual identity, and how she thinks others perceive her. Sophie described the experience of her sexual interaction with those in non-underrepresented groups as:

> **Sophie**: ...because of feeling marginalized by my orientation, I believe that as a creature, am sub-standard to have sex with. This means that I am lucky to get whatever I get from people I am choosing to be intimate with...this means reduced satisfaction in intimacy because of lack of advocacy for my preferences (due to reduced sense of self-worth, even though I have the power and safe space to self-advocate).

She discloses that the learned sense of unworthiness and lack of hope around trauma emerged at a young age:

> **Sophie**: um... just speaking of trauma which is where I originally learned like I'm not worth it and I can't do anything about it when I was like a teenager...

Similarly, Nathan discussed how the *individualized encounters with "isms"* by his perpetrator negatively impacted his self-worth:

> **Nathan**: ... yeah so I've often felt like my eyes been tied directly to my race, and I am now constantly aware that I'm short, and I have often felt very ashamed that I'm short, and I've been ashamed that I'm short because I'm Asian and it all tied to this one moment because before that I never really thought about how short I was

This shame has impacted his self-worth and he seems to consistently wonder whether he is good enough to belong to his current community. The intensity and impact of Nathan's negative *self-worth* was noticeable as Nathan worked to regulate himself through taking deep breaths and silence:

> **Nathan**: [tears & long silence] I guess to be told that you're short and just an Asian guy it's kind of like so that means that I am easily disposable or something and I do not know its [deep breath] ...[silence]

Similarly, Tim Samson discussed the ongoing and cyclical nature of the connection between body awareness and image and self-worth:

> **Tim Samson:** …it became a thing like I had to be attractive in order to be a good person and that's something I still like struggle with…. I'll go to the gym, and I'll work out, and I'm not doing it… I'm doing it half for health and half for vanity… and that vanity part is something that like I'm… it really, it's…. it's frustrating because I'm…. I know that it's not who I feel inside it's…. I'm still trying to like …like I have this idea in my mind, like 'if I go to [metropolitan city] like and I see any of those people, they are going to have this judgment towards me be like "what happened to [Tim Samson]? He used to be…"'

However, the realization that *self-worth* does not have to be associated with <u>body awareness and image</u> has helped Tim Samson shift his negative <u>self-worth</u> towards the positive. Tim Samson shared that joining a new profession that appreciates his presence as a human and promotes the idea of a whole self has contributed to the positive shift he has made:

> **Tim Samson:** …and of course, I was studying [previous profession] where it's all like 'What can you do? What can you do? What can you do? It wasn't like consider who you are…do do do… not… are are are…. I didn't have to be a unicorn.

On the other hand, in some ways, navigating life after sexual violence has created an insight to participants' values and the shift to advanced self-awareness:

> **Nathan:** yes, feeling guilty about how you might have been or who you might have been or views you may have held but… even though I felt guilty I was glad to be in a space where I was finally there was a clarity where this is what I shouldn't be, and this is what I should strive to be.

Nathan described the sexual violence as an "eye opening" experience that helped him develop an 'empathy' towards others who might be subjected to similar situations. He shared that he was able to be more "inclusive" in his thinking and actions, and has become more "emotionally responsive" both to himself and others. For example, Nathan describes values that he wants to adhere to:

> **Nathan:** I was capable of being introspective and reflective and kind of understanding 'there is a right and wrong way to act there is a way to present yourself to be in a relationship… there there's a particular way you should behave in a relationship and there is an openness that you need to consistently have with your emotions and your feelings and who you are' and its ultimately made me happier in that sense because

now that I am more emotional and I'm more open and I'm more willing to… to not be so close[closed] off. I found clarity…

Tim Samson also discussed the positive shift in his <u>self-worth</u> as his efforts to integrate trauma continue:

> **Tim Samson:** I'm …I'm finding that as the years go by and I sort of collect experiences both good, and bad, I have so much more autonomy in how I can define myself. I can define myself. It is not enough to say I am a good person because I am innocent, and nothing has happened to me so I might as well. It is… 'am a good person and I've survived these things, and I can carry them, and I can have compassion for other people with some degree of empathy.' With assault specifically but also just like life is challenging and things happen and so like taking it like: 'This bad thing happened to me that could be something that I just continue to have anger about and like and push away the world. Or, I could say this bad thing happened to me. This can become a superpower like I can …I can use. I can help my…my healing process can help inform the work I do to help others heal' and that just feels really good. I like I'm…. I'm really happy. I'm like the happiest I've ever been like…
>
> **Tim Samson:** and I like me so much better now because I know me better um yeah [tears of gratitude].

This realization and trauma integration that is connected to participants' <u>self-worth</u> also translated into how they view the world and create relationships with others:

> **Nathan:** and since then [sexual violence], I've just been on this kind of journey to better myself, to be better to people, to be better towards women, to be better towards just society as a whole, and to really be open to the struggles that all people face whether that's sexual struggles or economic struggles are…just always aware that people suffer.
>
> **Tim Samson:** It was like "I need you to like me. I need approval. I need, even if I'm [working with others], I need you to know that I'm trying my best. I'm a good [professional]…. ahhhaaa… me, me, me …" and I'm pretty able to decenter myself now.

Overall, participants discussed the role of positive <u>self-worth</u> in facilitating their process of trauma recovery. Negative <u>self-worth</u> related to their <u>body awareness and image,</u> such as body size and "derealization" during sexual encounters, added to the difficulty in the journey after sexual trauma.

Self-trust. The third dimension under the *subcategory* of *psychological responses* to sexual violence was self-trust. Trusting oneself was described by participants as the insight and ability to be present and feel grounded in their experiences and perception of the world. For instance, Nathan shared the constant self-questioning of whether he was sexually violated or *not*. Being able to trust himself about his ability to recall details has helped him to start the meaning-making process. In addition to Nathan, Nichole also discussed their ability to trust themselves, and the self-assurance that they deserve to be treated with respect:

> **Nathan:** …. I began to question [if sexual violence occurred] …maybe I'm leaving out details or maybe my memory is faulty or because you know that there's … I I've taken so many different psychology classes that have talked about how memory is faulty and that was something that I was always really concerned like maybe I'm just misremembering…but then I remembered the context of it [sexual violence] and I remembered how it wasn't a mutual exchange… it was something that happened, and I froze and tensed up…

> **Nichole:** yeah yeah yeah …um so I had so the internal response to the thing [sexual violence] was instead like 'I did not deserve that. this is not how people treat other people' like [laughter]…um I just yeah I …um knew …knew to respect myself and trust my perception of what had happened to me

Self-trust was also related to participants' ability to keep themselves safe and their ability to use their skills to secure their safety:

> **Christina:** Yeah. Yeah. I-I definitely trust it a lot more now, like the gut says no, gut says no, we're gonna get out of that situation. If I start to feel uncomfortable, I'm like, 'okay, where is that like exit plan?'

This experience of trusting one's "gut" was a significant tool for Christina to set her boundaries and assert herself when situations seem unsafe and unsecure. Christina also shared her tendency to hold back from trusting others:

> **Christina:** yeah. I still have very much that like boundary and figuring out like, 'okay, I am going to stay closed off until I know it's safe.' And even then, it's gonna be like a crack of the door open first, like dip your toe in the water. See if you can handle like one little thing…

> Christina: There have been times when I meet new people and like I will recognize a red flag; like I will recognize something I'm like 'oh, they're like interrupt'... This sounds weird... but like 'they're interrupting me when I speak so they're not really listening, so will they listen when I say no?' Like if 'you're not really listening because I was in the middle of a sentence, and you didn't notice. Then will you listen later on?'

Self-trust, like body awareness and image and self-worth, was described as an ongoing process:

> Christina: Yeah, absolutely it. It is a bit of both. Um, intuition with like making sure, sure that those boundaries are like kept when needed. And then also like when to set up some new ones. Like 'oh, I didn't realize that bothered me so much. We're gonna set that up now.... Let's not do that, or like maybe don't say those things because it's, it could be offensive to people or to me.'

Participants shared that self-trust has facilitated their experience of naming sexual violence as trauma, and has helped them ensure their personal boundaries are respected. This self-trust helped them to have a rich internal conversation that supports their recovery (?) process.

Self-talk. This is the fourth dimension under the *psychological response subcategory* discussed by participants as one of the major experiences following sexual violence. Participants disclosed both positive and negative conversations within themselves as they created meaning from their traumatic experience. Four participants discussed the importance of making a conscious and intentional decision to talk to themselves as they process trauma and/or any other challenges they may encounter in their lives:

> Christina: Oh, yeah, I talked to myself. I always check in with myself and like, figure out what I'm feeling before I try to get other people's opinions, because I know that there are times where I let their opinions and their emotions influence my own. And I don't need that.

> Nichole: (Long Pause) It's really-it's really mysterious, like I, um (pauses) I have a really developed internal dialogue with myself.

> **Nathan:** I was capable of being introspective and reflective and kind of understanding "there is a right and wrong way to act there is a way to present yourself to be in a relationship... there there's a particular way you should behave in a relationship and there is an openness that you need to consistently have with your emotions and your feelings and who you are."
>
> **Tim Samson:** Sometimes things hit and it hurts and like... I have enough perspective now in large part because of how I handled like this specific process [sexual violence] like to go... 'Is that a hurt hurt? Or is that like a hurt that I just have to take a nap?' like learning how to sort of like parse...through what steps to take after something sort of hits.

Moreover, two participants discussed their awareness and ability to differentiate negative from positive self-talk. This skill of differentiating the negative from the positive helped them to use self-talk as a coping skill rather than a detriment to their journey of healing:

> **Christina:** I really do try to be like careful about any negative self-talk. So just like focusing on that positive self-talk, like finding the little things to celebrate.
>
> **Nichole:** ...or is there something better you could do this time? Right, so (pauses) there are patterns that I have that are good ones and there are others that are just subconscious; you show habits. And there are some that are detrimental. So, umm (pause) um, yeah.
>
> **Nichole:** and I'm often like self-aware to a fault, right, for like, umm... (short pause) I realized after-after those two weeks like that it'd become a pattern...uhm mm... 'ok, this is the pattern you have started dressing differently to the studio; it's because you're feeling uncomfortable (short, uncomfortable laugh) being seen yadda yadda yadda psychoanalyzing myself; great. Cool. (Laughs)

Participants also discussed the deliberate decision to focus on positive self-talk to help them cope with challenging situations including triggers of sexual trauma:

> **Christina:** Yeah, so if I'm like saying that there's something positive within myself. I'm like, okay, yeah, like start doing a little bit more positive self-talk.
>
> **Nichole:** yeah totally ..um...I mean myself talk is just unrecognizable from what it was even four or five years ago ..

Participants disclosed that practicing intentional and positive self-talk has been helpful in managing the trauma responses following sexual violence.

Self-awareness. The fifth dimension under the *psychological responses subcategory* of **responding to trauma** was self-awareness, described by participants as an experience that allowed them to recognize *somatic responses, emotional responses* as well as *psychological responses* to sexual violence:

> **Christina:** because, after like… self-blame, I turn to anger, and then, realizing that that anger is just not useful …it's not like useful use of my energy, it's not productive. I don't need to be angry with the people around me if it's… no, like If I've healed [from sexual trauma] it shouldn't be affecting me so why be angry? Moving like from like learning from the book, kind of moving from self-blame or moving away from self-blame. But then noticing in myself, going towards anger, and then again going back to the book [Art of Happiness] and being like, okay? Well, what does he [the author] say about anger and then shifting into like, finally being at peace, and what I felt was like actually healed from that.

Participants discussed their effort to broaden their self-awareness so they can use their self-reflection to develop better strategies to cope with trauma and help them feel grounded in their positive self-worth. Below are Christina's thoughts on her self-awareness:

> **Christina:** yeah, exactly. yeah. figuring out like what I feel first and then going and talking to others.
>
> **Christina:** I have been described to be very insightful and very self-aware.

She recalled that she learned to be more *self-aware* and "check" with herself before inviting others into her world from observing others whom she perceived as being unable to be self-aware:

> **Christina:** So they're like you're just so self-aware and insightful like you're kind of set. I'm like 'cool. Thanks." Yeah. So I…I get that. But I do try to like [to] check in with… I think… I think part of that is seeing, and like from my past, other people not be self-aware…So I'm not gonna do that. So I'm gonna be hyper aware of myself.

For Christina, there is a process of self-preservation from disclosing *emotional and somatic responses* related to any life challenges before weighing in on the pros and cons. It seems that she made a conscious decision to carry the weight of being "hyper" aware to protect herself and others:

> **Christina:** ...so I have had to make like the active, active decision to be like, 'No, we're processing this. We're gonna think everything through.' If I'm mad in the moment I'm gonna move myself away. Process it. See if I'm still mad. See if it's actually worth it [to disclose]. Come forward with like a plan to discuss. Like it...it's a whole process, but it came from like seeing other people not do that [be self-aware], and then feel like seeing how it made me feel. And then being like, I don't want that for I don't want to make anyone else feel like that.

Participants also talked about the unintended negative outcomes of self-awareness despite its benefit in processing traumatic experiences:

> **Christina:** I think that self-reflection and just actually getting to know who you are is very important in the healing process. And it's something that's really hard and not fun. Because once you get to know yourself, sometimes there's things that you really don't like.
>
> **Tim Samson:** [self-awareness is] lovely and its intimidating it's... it's scary to become self-aware. It is like.... you have to take the good with the bad
>
> **Nichole:** I'm often like self-aware to a fault, right, for like...

Despite these negative emotions related to self-awareness, most participants shared the positive outcomes of self-awareness. Moreover, their experience of self-awareness and comparing their values of pre and post trauma has helped participants to develop more *empathy* for others who might be suffering.

Empathy. The sixth dimension under the *subcategory* of *psychological responses* was empathy, described as the conscious shift to relate to others after experiencing sexual trauma. Participants shared that some of their empathy is for those with similar sexual violence experience because they can recognize the hurt at a deeper level. For others, it is a general recognition that people suffer, and this leads them to be more empathic to others around them. For instance, Nathan talked about his ability to relate to other sexual violence and trauma survivors after having experienced the same, while Nichole shared their ability to relate to other survivors emotionally:

> **Nathan:** I feel like… I can just relate to other people and I feel like it [sexual violence] has made me more empathetic towards a lot of the struggles that… that all people go through and especially women like that's why I would hate to feel misogynistic because it's opened my eyes to just how serious this [sexual trauma] is and how dehumanizing an experience like this [sexual trauma] can feel to where you feel like an object.
>
> **Nichole:** when this happened to me I …um thought of all like my friends who had voiced similar experiences to me with whom I could not at the time empathize you know, and I became angry for them too.
>
> **Nichole:** … um I wanted to like … it feels more authentic to open myself up to the pain of others than… um …to shut it out or ignore it too… I do not know…it's hard to explain.

Other participants talked about their ability to connect with others and to develop an altruistic mindset of helping others who may have experienced traumatic and/or sociocultural struggles similar to their own:

> **River:** And that was a thing for me that was like 'I'm making a choice but they're [queer adolescents disowned by their parents after coming out and living on the street] not.' And I think that really framed, especially when I was that young, I think it really framed it to be like, 'well if I ever get a chance, I wanna help but if these type kids that think they don't have anywhere to go.'
>
> **River:** and I'm like well maybe if I get good enough at it [earning money] I can help other people like, you know, because that was I mean that definitely be a good goal for me is just like, write a book just saying, just laying myself out there and just being like well one person can gain something, then that's a victory yeah so.
>
> **Sophie:** another thing that I think makes it [the healing process] kind of clunky is secondary trauma from working with clients….yeah, I don't, yeah, I don't know if it's triggered or it's their trauma that I'm just, you know, just, yeah, I don't know if I even would have needed to have my own experience to absorb theirs.

Participants reported that they started to experience more empathy towards those who might be potentially subjected violence and oppression. There strengthened their altruistic self and engaged in advocating for themselves as others because of their new understanding of trauma.

Naming and normalizing. This dimension of naming and normalizing emerged under the *subcategory* of *psychological responses* described by participants as one of the key components in the journey after experiencing sexual violence. Several participants shared the power of naming the sexual trauma, their identities and its intersection as well as gaining a diagnosis as a step forward.

Naming traumatic experiences, including sexual violence, was associated with participants' insights into the personal responses to their trauma and helped them to create an awareness around the situation. For some participants, the naming of the traumatic experience was a shock that marked the beginning of their journey of healing:

> **Tim Samson:** …I started talking about those instances in those events. She [therapist] was just like "I am going to stop you for a second here" [gesture of blocking] What you're describing is is A) assault and B) the way you are describing it, it sounds like it traumatized you. And, and that hit me like a freight train.
>
> **Nathan:** [deep breath] accepting that it [sexual violence] happened coz when it first happened I kind of… I remember the night that first happened I kind of went home and I wasn't certain if it had actually happened or if I had imagined it… you know what I mean like… it was kind of like one of those moments like "did that really happen"?"

Similarly, River shared the role that the #MeToo movement played in naming the sexual encounters as rape. This naming has helped River to clarify the confusion around trauma responses:

> **River:** Like obviously I wish this [sexual violence] wouldn't have happened, and I wish I would have been able to name it at the time, I think that definitely would have saved me a lot of just, like, inner pain from a place I didn't know why it hurt.

Reflecting back, two participants noticed how they handled the responses to traumatic experiences before they were able to name the trauma as sexual violence:

> **Tim Samson:** …this was until 2 years ago I was seeing a counselor we were just walking through like I have a lot of anger about my career, and I was like 'I do not really get it.' I was having a hard time finding the source of it… I was unaware how traumatic it [sexual violence] was for a long time.
>
> **Nathan:** …. I think…. so, the incident happened and then I didn't talk about it I acted like nothing happened.

The shift from denial and confusion about the sexual trauma to naming it has helped participants with trauma integration:

> **Tim Samson:** …able to name it like you said like by I experienced something that had a bad impact on me. and I have been like hiding it for a long time.

Naming also helped River to develop the skills to contain the negative emotional, somatic, and psychological responses to trauma:

> **River:** and then once…it's like once I was able to name it, it was almost like I was able to shrink it. Because I was able to you know kind of put it in a box, instead of it being like the thing was just floating inside of me; it's in a box, pad lock on it. Like it's there; I recognize that it's there, but it doesn't hold me back.

Through the experience of naming the nonconsensual sexual encounter as traumatic, participants were able to accept that the sexual violence occurred to them. One participant discussed the internal conversation of naming their experience as sexual violence, reporting that this had helped them to accept the event and move on to address it:

> **Christina:** with the first one. It was really coming to terms with what happened like really realizing that 'this happened to me that…' I was like 'it now just wasn't like a story that you hear like as a warning as like before I came to college…I identified as female so, or as a woman so like as a girl coming to college like you hear the…all the warning stories. I never thought it would actually happen to me. So, the first one I was really just like coming to terms with like "I experienced that. And now what?"

Accepting the sexual violence as a traumatic event helped participants to reframe the meaning they gave to the event and focus on the process of integrating trauma into their journey.

Naming and accepting has helped participants realize that the sexual encounter(s) was sexual violence:

> **Nathan:** ...and the more that I accepted that it did happen the more that like I continuously had these images in my head of what happened, and I came to terms with "yes this happened to me" and I ultimately didn't like it.... not ultimately ... I didn't like it and see the reason why I say that is because there was a time where I was like maybe... maybe I asked for it.
>
> **Tim Samson:** "This bad thing happened to me that could be something that I just continue to have anger about and like and push away the world. Or, I could say this bad thing happened to me. This can become a superpower like I can ...I can use. I can help my... my healing process can help inform the work I do to help others heal."

Participants also discussed how they noticed that the naming and accepting helped them transition to normalizing. Some of these normalizing experiences are self-initiated and involve the hard work participants themselves have done to learn more about what it means to experience sexual trauma:

> **River:** umm I mean I guess really the #MeToo movement.... I feel like that was probably the biggest thing because it allowed me to identify it. and in that I was you know able to start like healing and talking about it and coming to terms with it and, so yeah, I feel like that was a big moment just because it, like one I was like 'OK well I'm definitely not alone,' which I always kind of knew because like you know I have friends with stories but it was like it just reframed it in a way so that my experience felt valid for what I think my subconscious had already identified it with but I was able to like consciously identify it and I felt like that was really important.
>
> **Nathan:** I do take comfort in knowing that I'm not the only person out there who has faced this and while it's often an issue that is gendered in a lot of social circles I do feel like I can relate to others who have experienced it, and when I'm able to open myself up to those feelings and know that this is something that has happened to so many others.
>
> **Nathan:** ...I think that that this [sexual violence] particular issue because this particular issue is something that can happen to anyone.

Another participant talked about his efforts to impart information to the next generation by normalizing that anyone on the gender spectrum could be subjected to sexual violence, and by imparting knowledge and wisdom about consent:

> **Tim Samson:** yeah, even like been able to share it with my son. And he was like, I thought important, I did not like obviously go in detail with him but it was like "This is something. I think that, as we are talking about, we talk about consent, he started to be interested in girls, we are, well okay well.

Authenticity. One *property* that emerged under the *subcategory* of *psychological responses* to **responding to trauma** was *authenticity*. The experience of *authenticity* was described as the experience of feeling comfortable in presenting oneself to the society with congruence. Participants talked about the overarching role of *authenticity* in that it encompasses their ability to freely express themselves and their identity. Three participants talked about their *authenticity* and its connection with their happiness:

> **Nathan:** exactly like for example my hair is green and two years ago I would have never done my hair a...a funky color like this but after reading these books and thinking I should just be whoever I wanna be because people who are who they are ..are happier I had this confidence to just kind of "I'm gonna dye my hair..i am gonna wear colors like pink... I'm gonna pull off these styles and I don't think that affects my masculinity at all.

> **River:** So, I felt like "well if I could just be authentic with things and like people won't have to like question me. they'll just take me as I am." And then like the older I get the more I'm just like "let it all hang out. I'm like whatever this is me. I'm an open book, like, take me as... you want to... like you know if you don't like me, we don't have to be friends like you know it's I never saw the need to like hide parts of myself because all I really want is, just like in like making friends and relationships, all I want is like for people to know who I am as a person and if I have to hide parts of that then it's not honest and it's not real.

> **River:** you know, it's like it's because- I just see that- it's like I don't- one; I'm a terrible liar so I don't even bother anyway (laughter) and two; it's like I never saw the point it's like why you just have to make more excuses. so, I felt like being authentic was kind of my only option.

Authenticity also referred to the integration and congruence of the work participants have done on themselves in making meaning of their past experience, recognizing their present experiences, and hoping for the future. Tim Samson, for instance, discussed the peaceful nature of presenting oneself *authentically*:

> Tim Samson: I mean I've had rougher patches since then. It's not like living on this [smooth] like.... But there are moments where I'm like... I'm living and sitting with my memories and living and sitting with my history. I'm living and sitting with my hopes, and they do not feel like they are in conflict. They can be in the same room.

Based on the participants' experiences, *authenticity* was related to their understanding of self as well as the congruence between their identity and identity expression.

The *psychological responses* to trauma, characterized by dimensions of body awareness and image, self-worth, self-trust, self-awareness, empathy, self-talk, and naming and normalizing, and a *property* of *authenticity*, constituted participants' intentional and concentrated efforts to shift negative thoughts to positive ones. Participants also shared the relatedness of the properties under this *subcategory*. The following *subcategory, behavioral responses,* shows participants' efforts to translate these *psychological responses* into healing skills and practices.

Behavioral responses. The fourth *subcategory* that emerged within the **category** of **responding to trauma** was *behavioral responses.* This *subcategory* represents the actions participants engaged in to address their responses to the trauma and to positively transform their experience after sexual violence. Some of these immediate *behavioral responses* were negative experiences that participants disclosed as they tried to put themselves out into the world following the sexual violence experience. Nichole, for instance, disclosed how they dressed to protect their body from others around them:

> Nichole: I remember the first 2 1/2 weeks after the incidents, I was, like, dressing differently. I wouldn't show up to the studio without a shirt anymore. I mean I would up until that point I was just coming in the sports bra and the biker shorts, no problem, and then after that [sexual violence] I was like T-shirt, long leggings, keep on... keep my sweater on or something. I just felt like, so uncomfortable being seen as if like someone could tell that I'd been assaulted.

Nichole also talked about the shift in physical space and boundaries on touch that needed to be adjusted after the experience of sexual violence:

> **Nichole:** And I also didn't allow my teachers to adjust me [in yoga practice] for a long time.

The *subcategory* of *behavioral responses* was supported by five *properties* that indicate the types of behavioral engagements participants selected to help them deal with the sexual trauma. These *properties* are *knowledge acquiring, body movement, journaling and writing, therapy,* and *physical distance from the perpetrator.*

Knowledge acquiring. This *property* refers to participants' effort to educate themselves about trauma responses and obtain general knowledge about victims and survivors of sexual trauma. One participant discussed reading a book to learn and practice skills for a happier life:

> **Christina:** lot of my healing actually was because I did research on like the brain and fight or fight responses, and also like kinda how the brain works in situations like this. I intellectualized it all...so I stuck my nose in psychology books, and actually one book that really helped me in healing was the Art of Happiness...

Researching and finding potential explanations of *somatic responses* to trauma have been helpful for Christina to address the challenges of repeated sexual violence experiences. On the other hand, Nathan talked about the importance of educating himself about the suffering of women from sexual violence because, after his experience with sexual violence, he was better able to relate to their suffering:

> **Nathan:** and I started reading a lot more... just different... just different books really and I started to learn more about like struggles that women have gone through because I realized that as a man, I had to be a positive member of community ...

This effort to learn more about women's struggles in society was related to the shift in Nathan's values and his interest in becoming an inclusive and helpful member of society. For both Christina and Nathan, learning about trauma and trauma responses have been helpful in creating awareness of self and others.

Body movement. The second *property, body movement,* refers to participants' efforts to engage in physical activity that they found to be helpful in addressing their responses to trauma. One of the participants shared that doing yoga has been paramount in their healing journey. The participant described yoga as a tool to connect within their body and their spirituality, and had become a way of life rather than just a coping skill:

> **Nichole:** something that felt like a spiritual practice, and it just so happened also be this physical activity …um…ah…moving meditation so …um…that has been essential to my life in [town].

> **Nichole:** yoga practice changed my life seriously I like um I can't imagine who I would be right now if not for that and it wasn't even that long ago…

In addition, other participants shared the value of *body movement* through physical activities. When describing the healing moments, Sophie shared the role that outdoor therapy has in her healing journey:

> **Sophie:** another big piece that I didn't feel like healing in the moment but retroactively is, yeah, is a lot of the do a lot like outdoor therapy is my jam and that is a situation where your body is what you've got to work with and reliably shows up for you if you take care of it and you take safe risks…

> **Sophie:** um…. some mindfulness pieces I think that I've learned I of…why do I know that I'm safe right now? … I have bear spray with me…I know that the people around me are other mental health workers who I have hired. I know that the kids are safe, or I wouldn't have allowed them to be …. sometimes I try to remind myself like that was that was then versus now …

Body movement, mainly hiking and yoga, have helped participants create a spiritual connection with nature and their body respectively. This increased their body awareness as well as identity exploration.

Journaling and writing. The third property under the *subcategory* of *behavioral responses* was *journaling and writing*. Three participants discussed the benefit of using journaling and other writing opportunities to express their hurt and experience with sexual trauma:

> **Christina:** Everything just emotions, thoughts, but just brain dump in a journal, and sometimes go back and read it, and then try to figure out like, what did I mean here when I said, that emotion made me feel like a cactus like, like what? What does that mean?
>
> **Nichole:** ... I have poems that like, well I don't think they were inspired in the positive way but they, um, they only exist because the thing [sexual violence] happened and so I think in a way, although they're not like about that, they're-they come from it or are about it, on a subconscious level.
>
> **River:** So it's like help me go through like the cycle of memories, which is just really interesting and I feel like, because I have written a little bit about like (pause) uh, my experiences like rape and sexual assault and I feel like every time I do it, it's like, it's like getting it out of my insides and putting it somewhere else and it-it feels good but you know I don't share with anyone. it's still like feels...

Although Christina, Nichole and River talked about the private nature of their writing as "a brain dump" and "getting it out of my insides", Nathan discussed his experience of using poetry as a tool to disclose what has happened to him:

> **Nathan:** I had a poetry professor who wanted us to write about something personal there are poetry, and I wrote about it [sexual violence] and why... don't think the poem was is particularly good and...she felt that it was interesting that I talked about it [sexual violence] and I said... I told her that she was the only person outside of my partner [who] heard about it.

As a result, *journaling and writing*, whether as a course assignment or "cathartic" outlet to emotions, was found to be a helpful tool in the participants' journey.

Therapy. The fourth *property* under *behavioral responses* was *therapy*. Participants discussed the benefit of therapy in developing <u>self-awareness</u> and in their trauma recovery:

> **Tim Samson:** ...I started talking about those instances in those events. She [therapist] was just like "I am going to stop you for a second here" .... I did EMDR one time...

> Christina: ...with a therapist, and just actually let myself cry and have my therapist be like Where do you feel that in your body? and like actually being like whoa in my body? what? we feel emotions in our body? and then be like I feel it in my chest or in my stomach. That was very helpful because I actually let myself feel things like I wasn't just intellectualizing at all. And I wasn't going to do that by myself. I needed someone around me to basically validate my emotions so that I could validate them myself.

> Sophie: yeah, those are some things I'm trying to think of other healing um...therapy has been great, yeah, I mean I think of that being validated as a human helps us feel safer in our own bodies for sure.

In addition to increasing *self-awareness, therapy* helped participants to name and receive validation and support rather than questioning when they disclosed their experience of sexual trauma.

Physical distance from the perpetrator. The fifth and final *property* under **behavioral responses** and **responding to trauma** was participants' desire and continuous effort to have a *physical distance from the perpetrator*. Participants shared their fear of seeing their perpetrator in the community, and struggled with the uncertainty of how they would react in those situations:

> Nichole: it remains a little bit challenging wondering if I'll run into him again in town I think if and... and there was there was a long time where that kept me from going out to places um and I still try not to show up to things by myself just you know like and that's not because I feel like I couldn't set a boundary like I wouldn't like go talk to him or anything [laughter].

> River: went back to like see my family and like go to a show with my friends and that... the person was still working at the show venue, he was even the general manager, which just made me roll my eyes, and I totally saw him, we totally ignored each other and but like the whole time that I was supposed to be, like, enjoying this show of one of my favorite bands I was thinking about that bastard that was walking around.

Nichole disclosed their perception of sharing a physical space with the perpetrator following the sexual violence.

> Nichole: um... the person ... my aggressor was a housemate and when it [sexual violence] happened we're not quite moving out, but we were about to so there were four weeks where, I knew that I would be out of this situation, and there wasn't really any further action I could take to not be around them ...
>
> Nichole: um... [silence]...so I just I just kind of needed the time to pass and I spent as much time as possible not the house. [It] was really predictable when he would be there [at the house] ...yeah.... uhm... I ended up staying .... I never ...I didn't stay the night at all that month but like needed to be there to like pack and clean the house and [somber silence] yeah... it was bad [laughter].

Another participant shared their decision to maintain *physical distance* from their perpetrator and hoped their decision would be supported by their friends as well:

> River: ...yeah there are and it's like I've come to terms with person one and then, and I think it's a big thing because obviously none of my friends talk to him anymore, and but person two is still someone I have friends that are friends with. And one of my friends gave the excuse of "oh, well he's lonely and doesn't like have any friends" I'm like "there's a reason for that" ... I was like "don't feel bad for him" and uh...

Both Nichole and River shared their desire to avoid a physical encounter with their perpetrator following the sexual violence. However, as supported by Nichole's experience, not seeing their perpetrator may not always be possible. Another participant shared that their privacy and physical distance were interrupted due to social media algorithms. Sophie shared that she was "triggered" when Facebook proposed her perpetrator as "people you may know."

> Sophie:...um...Facebook recently said 'people you may know' and I see this person's face [the perpetrator] for the first time in 20 years who I've been having nightmares about for the last 20 years...and that was so dysregulating because one of the things I tried to tell myself to make myself feel safe is 'I live across the country from that person'...there's a huge [physical distance] ...and then Facebook like....and I felt like 'Oh my God he can get me' just like that reaction that...

She further elaborates on the lack of control as a survivor of sexual violence resulting from social media algorithms that minimize the sense of safety due to a narrowing of perceived distance from the perpetrator:

> Sophie: yes, I think social media now can constantly keep these people or if you want to cut off that person you can't necessarily do that...

> Sophie: 'can he look me up and see my' you know or whatever, so I think there is that feeling vulnerability with.... with social media that adds to it that I don't get to control, right, and his access to me which is .... takes us right back to right the beginning...that I don't get to control his access to me...

In general, participants' *behavioral responses* have shown their effort to find ways that help them manage the negative experiences following sexual violence.

Participants shared their experience of **responding to trauma** as filled with *somatic responses, emotional responses, psychological responses,* and *behavioral responses*. Each of these subcategories of responding to trauma had both negative and positive implications. Participants also disclosed their relationship with **the perpetrator** as well as the perpetrator's identity as they reflected on their journey of **responding to trauma**.

The Perpetrator

Another theme that emerged based on participants' experience after sexual violence related to their views about **the perpetrator**. This **category** refers to the participants' perceptions and encounters with the perpetrator that impacted their journey following sexual violence in mostly negative ways. There are two *subcategories* under this **category**: *the perpetrator's identity* and *perpetrator's attempt to contact the survivor* after the sexual violence.

The perpetrator's identity. This *subcategory* explains the power and privilege the perpetrator held prior to committing the sexual violence. Tim Samson shared that the power and privilege of one of his perpetrators was intertwined with his aspiration to become a performer. He disclosed getting a reward from the perpetrator that provided a distraction from focusing on the sexual violence:

> **Tim Samson:** and it became part of how I got cast, you know, ... this one [person of power], who had a lot of power in the community... he had a lot of....He was very

attracted to me, and he would often just find ways of [me] being [in] his [professional engagements], and like, you know, there's a big [professional role] or not like I would just, you know, my bargain worked.

The perpetrator's power and authority were also factors in River's experience of witnessing and being subjected to sexual violence at the hands of the police. This later determined River's decisions not to report sexual violence and a preference to avoid possible interactions with the justice system:

> **River:** 'ok, I guess that's just how they [the cops] treat women'... that was kind of just like 'ok, I'm gonna do everything in my power to stay away from them [cops] now.'

Another participant also discussed the privilege of the perpetrator in relation to his race and familiarity with the community where the sexual violence happened:

> **Nichole:** my aggressor was a white man who has lived in [town] his whole life probably yeah just like has a lot of he's... he does sweet talks about any basically anything.

The systemic and ongoing transgressions Nichole experienced as a gender nonbinary and queer person of color contributed to the biases they have towards anyone who shares the perpetrator's racial identity. As Nichole noted:

> **Nichole:** I do have like dear friends who are not that person...but about whom I still make assumptions based on my exper[iences]- past experiences with white men, right? So, it's just, um (pauses) yeah maybe that's the end of the thought. I know that there's work to do there yeah... I would just like one of them to prove me wrong (laughs).

In the same vein, Nathan, whose perpetrator was a white woman, stated that his anger and resentment were directed to women -- especially educated women -- whom he perceives as dismissive of men's sexual trauma survivor's experience:

> **Nathan:** ...um...I started to become increasingly resentful towards women and that was because I started to see that women at the school don't think particularly highly of men at least in my experience.

Two participants disclosed experiencing acts of sexual violence from both male and female perpetrators. These participants shared their negative reactions and caution as they interact with others who identify as men following their sexual violence encounter. For instance, Christina, who identifies as both bisexual and queer, stated that the sexual violence experience not only provided some clarity about her sexual orientation but also contributed to the generalized fear towards men:

> **Christina:** ... how I felt about myself between the first and the second event like between those 2, the second event I knew that was not my fault for a 100% sure...mmhmm...that was not a question. Uh-uh! Being like no! this makes me 100% sure about my sexuality like men? no! They are no! ... Even though I didn't want to, for the women, like I was like 'No, that's just like one in a 1 million.' For the men I was like 'that's all of them like cut n[and] dry.' I let that like very much set in my brain.
>
> **Christina:** Oh, yeah. yeah, I'm cautious with everyone, but especially with men. mostly because of the size difference.

Similarly, for Tim Samson, who disclosed that he had experienced "multiple" sexual violence incidents from "both men and women", the fear for safety is primarily associated with individuals who identify as gay:

> **Tim Samson:** That's why feel like I would... I would have a really hard time being around like outwardly gay men. And like. And, why, what? I don't have like...there's no philosophical challenge there. It's just like 'oh, this is the population that like if I get around you, you're probably going to do something that is kind of damaging my sense of safety."

In sum, the above voices show the intersection of sexual violence with the **sociocultural contexts** of the survivors of sexual trauma. The authority and the power and privilege the perpetrator held had influenced participants' responses to the trauma as well as their decisions to seek justice.

Perpetrator's attempt to contact the survivor. The second *subcategory* under the **perpetrator** was *perpetrator's attempt to contact the survivor*. Two participants talked about their confusion about the why and how of the attempt to contact them. Christina recalled receiving a call from one of her perpetrators who made no attempt to recognize the wrongdoing and/or apologize:

> **Christina:** Yeah, as if nothing happened. And so, I think that also like sat with me wrong. Like how could you just pretend that nothing happened? Realizing that that was something huge for me? But maybe just like another Saturday for them like. Yeah, so that would that one was very... I was not doing well after that. I had to like, I felt that I had to, almost, like restart that healing process of being like, huh, if they're so okay with it, then was it really my fault? No. It wasn't!
>
> **Christina:** No. Nothing [no apology]. Just like "Hey!" Hey. Exclamation point... like it's all good like "how is it that like? How are you? How's it going?" Hey? Like no, not exactly like... who? who in the right mind would do that, right?

Another participant also shared their confusion around the attempt of the perpetrator to talk to them after the act of sexual violence:

> **Nichole:** just kept trying to talk to me I just like I couldn't understand why. There's just so much... I just could not understand why he was trying to talk to me [laughter, facial expressions and body gestures showing confusion].

Christina recalls getting triggered and dysregulated due to the *perpetrator's attempt to contact the survivor* to the point that her *somatic responses* were visible to her friends. She stated that the lack of safety she felt during the brief phone conversation she had with the perpetrator was restored after her friends intervened to take measures to set boundaries on her behalf:

> **Christina:** After that, like they [friends] took my phone, and they blocked that person on like everything that they could like, tried like even went to go find them on extra social media to block them to like 'you were not contacting. No, uh-uh. That is not happening anymore', and like deleted it off my phone, make sure that it was like all gone. She [friend] was like "look, I'm even Clorox wiping your phone. It's like all gone."

In general, the participants in this study talked about their desire to create a *physical distance with the perpetrator*. They also shared the triggers around the *perpetrator's attempt to contact them* especially when the attempt was without recognition of the wrongdoing. Participants also shared the intersection of the perpetrator's sociocultural context and identity with theirs and noted that this intersection influences their responses to trauma and decision-making. Participants also shared that the power and privilege related to *the perpetrator's identity* influenced their experiences and perspectives towards **the perpetrator** and those who share similar identities.

Disclosure

The sixth major theme participants discussed was **disclosure**. The **category** of **disclosure** is defined by the participants' experience of sharing their violent sexual encounters with others, their reasons for disclosure, and the outcomes of the disclosure. Participants shared that their experience of being questioned or having to justify their claims of having been sexually violated added to the hardship after the trauma. However, the experience of getting validation, normalization and space-holding as participants disclosed their experience to others contributed to a more positive outcome and facilitated their trauma integration process.

Three participants discussed the benefit of disclosure as a significant factor that facilitated positive outcomes in their journey after experiencing sexual trauma:

> **Tim Samson:** talking about it! talking about it! talking about it! Um... name it to tame it or whatever.
>
> **Nathan:** one of the things that I feel that has helped me move past it [sexual trauma] or like kind of put it [sexual trauma] behind me is talking about it.
>
> **Christina:** Yeah, I feel like the best way to de-stigmatize this [sexual trauma] and actually get some change is to talk about it. So, I've gotten comfortable with that.
>
> **Christina:** I'm a verbal processor. So whenever, like. If someone's like, tell me about your day, it's great, because then I can actually like, think about my day and like, go

through it. So, being able to start to talk to people about like what happened, I actually started to be like, okay, that actually happened. I'm healing. I'm processing that.

However, the process of **disclosure** was also challenging for some participants. Two participants discussed the difficult nature of disclosure and discussions involving sexual violence and trauma:

> **Nichole:** Yeah, it was hard, it was hard because (pause) at um, (pause) there's like no… there's no soft way to enter that conversation and like you can't …lead up to it anyway.
>
> **Nathan:** and it's [talking about sexual violence and disclosing] been a struggle and I'm still consistently trying to learn how to the proper way to really articulate my feelings in a way where the point gets across and everyone understands …and everyone learns a little bit differently so finding a common ground among all people is as kind of been my goal.

Therefore, Nichole needed to switch their approach of communication into formal conversation and provide a warning that they are about to disclose something significant:

> **Nichole:** the first thing that I said was "Hi I'm about to say something really serious," and that kind of helps. She and I both shift in order to make room for the weight of that conversation. Um, it also made sure that I wasn't diminishing the weight of it in any way, that both knew we were there for our conversation at that point, so that helped.

Disclosure has two *subcategories* that explain the personal considerations and the interpersonal interactions participants experienced as they disclosed their sexual violence. These two subcategories are: *intrapersonal considerations of disclosure* and *interpersonal outcomes of disclosure*. Most of the *subcategories* and *properties* or <u>dimensions</u> under **disclosure** are marked as processes instead of experiences, showing movements from nonintentional disclosure to intentional disclosure determined by the outcomes of initial disclosures.

Intrapersonal considerations of disclosure. The *subcategory* of the *intrapersonal considerations of disclosure* refers to participants' experience of intentionality and goal of disclosure as well as their internal openness to receive support and engage in a conversation once they have disclosed their experience. The *subcategory* of *intrapersonal considerations of disclosure* is supported by one dimension: unintentional disclosure to intentional disclosure and a *property* of *purpose of disclosure*.

Unintentional disclosure to intentional disclosure. All six participants discussed their ability or lack thereof to control the parameters around disclosing their traumatic experience and its outcome. The control around disclosure was explained by participants' ability to be intentional about disclosing the sexual violence with the goal of either benefiting themselves or using their experience to educate and support others. Two participants shared that their experience of unintentional disclosure was intertwined with triggers. For these two survivors of sexual trauma, triggers accompanied by ongoing somatic and emotional trauma responses have forced them to disclose their sexual violence experience. Some of these physiological and psychological responses were, for instance in the case of Sophie, uncontrolled trauma responses:

> **Sophie:** my first sexual interaction with him [current partner] was something that happened with lots of people since my sexual trauma which is just this full on like just a panic attack like shaking, dissociation, hyperventilation, all that kind of stuff.
>
> **Nathan:** I wouldn't say that it [disclosure] was something that like I consciously and willingly did. It was more involuntary, and it just came out because I remember when it happened.
>
> **Nathan:** I was in an argument with my partner and then like as we were arguing, I just kind of broke down and it just came out [disclosure of sexual violence].

The transition from unintentional disclosure to intentional disclosure occurred with the participants' process of finding a purpose in their disclosure.

> **Nathan:** since then [the first disclosure] we've [participant and his partner] talked about it several more times and each time I've talked about it it's been in a less hostile way.

The remaining four participants discussed their internal process of decision-making as they intentionally disclosed their experience to trusted others. As they planned to share their sexual violence experience, participants attempted to find out how their disclosure would be handled. Two participants shared their efforts of disclosing sexual violence as if the experience was their friend's and/or some anonymous person:

> **Christina:** with my family, I didn't tell them out very...but I had shared with them...I was like, "oh, this happened to a friend of mine", not me, friend of mine... just kinda to gauge the reaction in case I did decide to tell them.
>
> **River:** I left me out of the question, and I was like "hey, so, let's say" ... I was like "do you consider this [nonconsensual sex] rape?"

Participants talked about their fear of disclosing the experience of sexual violence. The fear was associated with anticipating invalidating responses from those they disclosed to. This fear has prolonged their process of obtaining support. One participant talked about the personal healing journey she needed to go through before making an intentional decision to share her experience with her parents:

> **Christina:** yeah, and when it had first happened, I wasn't in a place to be judged like I knew mentally like the second they [participant's parents] judge me, it's all over... I like ...I will go downhill fast, so I waited until I had processed it. I had healed from it to then share with them.

As indicated in participants' process, the shift from <u>unintentional disclosure to intentional disclosure</u> has helped participants to decide the purpose of their disclosure of the sexual violence experience. Having control over when, how and to whom to disclose has been helpful for participants.

Purpose of disclosure. The *purpose of disclosure,* a *property* under the *subcategory* of *intrapersonal considerations of disclosures,* is explained by what participants plan to achieve by disclosing their experience of sexual violence. Two participants discussed their aim of changing others' perspectives or educating others about sexual trauma, while also discussing their intention to normalize the experience of sexual violence to other survivors:

> **Christina:** Yeah, I feel like the best way to de-stigmatize this [sexual trauma] and actually get some change is to talk about it. So, I've gotten comfortable with that.
>
> **River:** yeah definitely. Especially, like like I don't I always tell like my younger cousins too like I don't hold back from them just because I feel like the younger you know these things the better.
>
> **River:** it was like #MeToo movement happened and I felt like "wait, do I?... it's like now do I have something to say that might make other people that feel the same way as me feel differently and actually realize that what they went through is valid?"

The *purpose of disclosure* can also be intended to gain awareness and clarity in emotions and freely expressing them:

> **Christina:** by myself. I would just intellectualize all my emotions, not actually let myself feel. But when I was actually able to talk about it with friends or with a therapist, and just actually let myself cry.

As indicated in these participant voices, the *purpose of disclosure* was influenced by their intent to benefit others and help *name and normalize* the sexual violence experience. Overall, the experience of **disclosure** of sexual violence is portrayed by participants' effort to transition from <u>unintentional disclosure to intentional disclosure</u> in which the intentional disclosure informs their *purpose of disclosure*. All of these processes mark the intrapersonal considerations participants make before disclosing the sexual violence experience to others.

Interpersonal outcomes of disclosure. Another *subcategory* that emerged under the category of disclosure was *interpersonal outcomes of disclosure*. The *interpersonal outcomes of disclosure* are explained by the perceived social support upon disclosure. This subcategory also includes the experience of being questioned or blamed for disclosing sexual violence. Participants talked about the felt need to explain and justify the reasons for their conclusion that they have experienced sexual trauma. The *interpersonal outcome of disclosure* is supported by two *properties: social support* and *victim questioning.*

Social support. Participants stated that **disclosure** of their sexual violence to trusted others and its outcome changed the trajectory of their journey. Trusted others also provided corrective experiences in the form of *social support*:

> **Christina**: Yeah, if it wasn't for my best friend, I mean, I wouldn't be here today like she literally stopped me, and she's been with me through, 2 out of the 3 events. Or not like with me, but she's been there for me at the for 2 out of the 3 events, and like has supported me in school and work, and like all the areas of my life, and I have felt with her like more of unconditional love and like a better relationship, platonic relationship, but like a better and a more healthy relationship of like "I'm going to express my needs. And I'm going to listen to someone express their needs, and we're going to work through it." Like, actually have like a healthy relationship, that all happened with her. And so that definitely like having her, she was basically my saving grace.

> **Nathan**: my partner is very kind to me and my partner is white and she's always looked at me like I the most beautiful person in the world and that always makes me feel like I have value ..um...because I know that many people in life seek the kind of relationship that her and I have where we've been together for so long and we're very close friends and I... I mean that we're very close friends like we laugh together and we joke around together and we're so comfortable and natural with each other that it's strange to see one without the other.

They shared that the act of naming, validating and normalizing by others closest to them has positively facilitated their journey after experiencing sexual trauma. Participants discussed the different sources of *social support* which depended on the depth of vulnerability and trust established as they developed a sense of community. As a result, the *property* of *social support* has four *sub-properties:* sense of community and friendships, family support, support from romantic partners, and support from professionals.

Sense of community and friendships was discussed as a subcomponent of *social support* that helped participants to validate and normalize their experience. Three participants discussed the importance of having friends who were supportive, available and validating as they explored the meaning of their sexual violence experience:

> **Christina:** Yeah...my friends, some of my closest friends, and like they held you it or at least listen to me as I processed and cried about it.
>
> **Nichole:** and really developed sense of community and friendship [that helped in their journey], it just so happens that my cohort like jelled and like we made we found affinity with each other pretty quickly...yeah, and so it was hard to believe that [developing close friendship within short period of time] ...and not know what it was going to be [sense of community when moving to a new place] but out of that situation [rape] you knew really strongly what good friendship looks like when I saw it.
>
> **River:** I have this one friend she's basically my sister like [we] call each other sisters and she was immediately like "I knew there was something weird" she was like "I knew you never would have slept with him if you actually wanted to" but I was like "well you're the only one that thought that but thank you" like so she knew even though the language around it [consent] wasn't there.

Some friendship relationships have provided a sense of safety and served as a protective factor. One participant discussed in detail the role of a trusting close friendship in shielding her from self-harm following multiple sexual violence episodes:

> **Christina:** Yeah, if it wasn't for my best friend, I mean, I wouldn't be here today like she literally stopped me [dying by suicide], and she's been with me through, 2 out of the 3 events [sexual violence]...has supported me in school and work, and like all the areas of my life, and I have felt with her more of unconditional love.

This comfort in having a sense of community and friendship was not limited to the disclosure of sexual violence experience, but was also related to navigating life as a minority. One participant talked about the significance of a friendship group at a young age that was accepting of their identity, thus facilitating an authentic presence growing up:

> **River:** yeah so, it's like you know I was always pretty comfortable with the fact that I was queer especially in high school because I had a lot more queer friends... I was in drama um... and my friends were like really open and stuff.

Having a sense of community and friendships was also associated with an authentic presence for participants in which they felt accepted by those closest to them. One participant talked about the importance of *authenticity* in forming close friendships:

> **Tim Samson:** my friends. I mean one thing I will say, like I don't think I have any authentic friendships outside of my marriage until I came to [an educational program] that includes my previous grad school experience, like because I was never able to totally be me.

Another participant discussed the fear and hesitation to name his sense of community and friendship as a social support because the participant felt that they did not have the experience to name this friendship or community as a support system:

> **Tim Samson:** ... interesting that you say social support system, I feel fear saying that. I didn't name that as I was talking through it because I think I still feel like I don't have any friends. I have a ton of friends now and they're wonderful friends. But it's new...the relationships feel great, they feel stable, but yeah, I don't have enough history to say I have friends.

On the second *sub-property* of *social support,* participants talked about their family support. *Participants discussed that social support* was received from family members and relatives upon **disclosure** of experiences of sexual violence. For participants, **disclosure** to parents and parental figures was challenging. However, the outcome of validation and normalizing by family members facilitated a positive experience for participants as they continued life after sexual trauma:

> **Nathan:** another thing that keeps me going on is my brothers ... I'm the oldest of eight...but my two brothers who are from my dad... I'm very very close with them, and since we grew up within the same time frame and we live under a lot of the same experiences, we're very open with each other especially after I started to become more emotionally open to everyone.

> **River:** And my mom was, was like just like sat there. She likes to puzzle everything so she just started researching everything... she was like "I'm gonna read more about sexual trauma and I'm gonna read more about this" then I was like "ok, I think it was definitely transformative to them [mom and dad] because you know being older they saw it in a very different way.

> Tim Samson: Yeah. I'm really proud of being a parent. I love how much I love my kids and how I show up for them, so and you know, when I don't show up for them, it really helps me say "what is it that's making it so I can't show up for them?"

Another *sub property* under *social support* was support from romantic partners. Support from romantic partners was also discussed as a significant factor that contributed to feeling grounded as participants disclosed their sexual violence experience, both intentionally and unintentionally:

> River: I told my partner. I've been with him for almost 14 years now, and he was like... he just like gave me a hug and he's like "anything I could do?" and I'm like just be you, like, "thank you."

> Tim Samson: I feel really insulated and protected by my marriage...when I told her [my wife] [about the sexual trauma] ...when I was seeing that counselor that helped me sort of parse this all out. I was like I came home, and I told her about it and "oh my god, it makes total sense" ... and "thank you for telling me this." She was really warm about it.

> Sophie: I regulate better when I'm being squeezed... we did not know each other for long... but for him luckily he was able to read the situation and just kind of held me tight which for someone else could have been the very wrong thing to do but for me it happened to be the right thing to do and then that was kind of a switch for me where I was like "ok, this is safe."

> Sophie: so that that helped to as a verbal processor to feel not just like tolerated but like accepted and seen and still wanted.

> Nathan: where she's [partner] kind of like "I wanna know more because I want you to talk about this" and I've been able to talk about it and reflect on it and articulate it in a way where I feel like I've become more open to her, and she's been more open to me and we both see each other's feeling.

The last *sub property* under *social support* was support from professionals including peers and colleagues. Two participants discussed the importance of support from the professional group they joined:

> Tim Samson: and of course, I was studying [previous profession] where it's all like...What can you do? What can you do? What can you do? It wasn't 'consider who

you are.' At least my experience is do do do not are are are... then moving to a place where I was approved of in a very specific way.

Nathan: I work at the [middle] school. I am a substitute teacher there. It's a little community and I really like that since it is such a progressive learning area like everyone's really really close knit tight, everyone knows everyone... and being around kids makes me happy... because it challenges my thinking and it forces me to see the world as they might see it.

Overall, the perceived *social support* from parents, partners, friends, professionals, and community helped participants engage in a positive journey after sexual trauma. *Social support* was also a significant factor that helped participants authentically express their identities and in turn contributed to the positive journey following sexual violence.

Victim questioning. On the other hand, the questioning, blaming, and invalidating upon disclosure in some cases added to the difficulty of the journey after sexual trauma. Three participants shared their negative experiences regarding this *property, victim questioning*, and one participant expressed this fear of being questioned as limiting their desire to share their experience with significant others:

Nathan: um...in the process of healing I think that the most difficult things has been... I often feel invalidated um...by, and I hope this doesn't come across misogynistic, but ...by a lot of women specially here on campus because there's lots of talk about sexual assault all the time.

River: I started getting questions and like at that point I don't think I was ready for the questions... the second person, like, commented on that post and it was just like I... like looked at it and like immediately blocked them. I was like "Nope!"

River: Yeah, it's like so it's like am I overreacting? Am I, am I just jumping?... because, I got accused of like, "oh you're just jumping on the bandwagon of the #MeToo thing why didn't you say something before?" I was like "because I didn't know to process it before."

Christina: I had shared with them [parents] I was like... "oh, this happened to a friend of mine, not me friend of mine, just kinda to gauge the reaction" ...and it wasn't the reaction that I wanted or expected. It was a little bit more negative, a little bit more like victim blaming, asking, "well, what was she wearing? What did she do?" and hearing that from them was... it was difficult. It was very difficult to process that.

> **Nathan:** one of the books that we're discussing focused around sexual assault, and I remember that the women in my class began to talk about it... they gendered it a lot... they made it so it was...it was... it was "what we had to teach men to not do this."

As indicated in participants' statements in the **disclosure category**, some participants shared that they were questioned and invalidated instead of getting support, adding to the complexity of their journey after sexual trauma. Participants' *intrapersonal considerations of disclosure* incorporate the process of a shift from unintentional disclosure to intentional disclosure. Often this shift to intentionality helped clarify the *purpose of disclosure* for participants. Once **disclosure** was made, the outcome was either *social support* or *victim questioning*. *Victim questioning* often triggered and added to the negative recovery journey from sexual trauma. On the other hand, the support from significant others was associated with feeling validated. Validation and normalization of the experiences of sexual trauma have helped participants to experience moments of safety, relief, and empowerment.

Moments of relief and empowerment

The seventh **category** to emerge based on the participants' experience was **moments of relief and empowerment**. This **category** refers to the specific events or sets of events that helped participants feel safe, secure, and free. Some participants shared specific events that informed them that there was light at the end of the tunnel. At the same time participants described the cyclical nature of the **moments of relief and empowerment**. To capture the range of **moments of relief and empowerment** from specific to general, I created a dimension of specific moments of relief to recognition of overall personal growth. Two participants describe the cyclical nature of trauma recovery reflected through the experiences of triggers that set off the **moments of relief and empowerment**:

> **Christina:** So, it yeah, definitely to start it off. It was very much like I felt like it was going well, and then, like something would happen, or I would remember something

have like a nice little flash back to what, the to the situation. And then I'd feel like I would go back to the beginning and like have to start over my healing process.

Christina: Yeah, I honestly would describe it as like a situation that felt like it was one step forward, 3 steps back, like it was very difficult to get through at first...I feel like, I'm constantly a work in progress now. But that's okay.

Nathan: um...you know it's difficult to articulate the process because a lot of times I..I often feel like I'm not entirely over it and simultaneously I am over it but like it's a part of me in the past but then there are sometimes where like I will lay awake at night now and I'll pop in my head and I'll think about it.

As participants reflected on their journey and recalled events that were connected with safety, assurance and security, they were able to recognize the importance of self-celebration and recognition of small everyday events. Two participants describe these experiences of safety and relief:

Christina: Yeah, any progress that's made is good progress, and one of my friends, she says, like, Yes, the big picture is important, but it's the small little details that like are award winning.... So it's the small little things like celebrate those. So yeah, and I really like, like, yeah, big picture is important. If you reach that big goal, Whoo! But, like those little, small ones, might be harder than that big one, or it might take longer to get past that tiny little one. So celebrate those.

Christina: yeah, so like anything that's like positive that I or that I'm working towards. And I see that I'm like, okay little treat, positive self-talk. You're doing great. Look at you go healing like; you didn't do the same thing as last time. Yay!

Nichole: So (pause) yeah I just like had gotten myself to a point where I was able to choose sexual activity for myself and which that was not the point for any of my life prior to that, so it almost felt like a response, not just to the incident, but to everything happened before that that felt like sexual repression and I could not- non choice, non-option. Um (pause) but yeah that was really, really intentional moment for me.

These moments can be associated with recognizing the progress they have made in becoming their authentic selves. Participants' **moments of relief and empowerment** ranged from specific moments of relief to recognition of overall personal growth. Some participants shared the collective meaning they ascribe to their sexual violence experience and ways in which they integrate trauma into the meaning they have made of their life:

> **Tim Samson:** Yeah, I'm a good person like "I like me and I like me so much better now because I know me better" um yeah... Thank you! [tearful] it feels good to say.
>
> **Tim Samson:** there are moments where I'm living and sitting with my memories and living and sitting with my history. I'm living and sitting with my hopes, and they do not feel like they are in conflict. They can be in the same room.
>
> **Nathan:** yeah and being really open with my feelings it has really just improved my relationships with people in general not just my partner but like friendships and relationships with my my my peers or coworkers or my professors like I've just been able to articulate like 'hey these are things that I'm not really happy with' not even regarding the just what happened but just in general it's just made me a a more emotionally available person
>
> **River:** because I...I was able to like view it from not the like masked part of myself but from like the actual part of myself and it was like out 'yeah it's ok to actually say out loud what happened to me was a rape even if I was drunk and even if you know I went into his room that doesn't you know even though I didn't verbally say no like that it's still you know my experience is still valid.'

For other participants the **moments of relief and empowerment** are clear visions of occurrences that they recall as reminders that healing is possible. These moments tell them that "it's gonna be okay."

> **River:** Honestly? I think kind of right now, because (laughter) because I'm (pause) like I'm not like pissed off right now, I'm not crying, I'm not like ranting, I'm like I feel like I'm at a place where I'm like 'yes, this is a thing that happened, it's important to talk about, I want people to know it's a thing that happened.'
>
> **Christina:** ...it was the night before my twentieth birthday....my two best friends from here in Montana, came to visit me, or went to visit me in Oregon, since I was home for a little bit in the summer, and I had definitely missed them like they were my support group here. They had been through it all with me.... we had gone to the beach earlier that day and came back home and the sun was setting. and we were at a park right by my house, and we took like a it's saltwater taffy that we got from the beach, and like some, some like some snacks like kind of a little picnic vibes and a blanket, and we went out to watch the sunset over the city, it's gorgeous, and so we turned on some like low-key music. It was very... it was so nice and like we were just like all dancing a little bit like just like kinda enjoying the time, and I felt really at peace. And then, right when, like the sun was setting, and it was about to get dark we laid down on the blanket, and it was one of my friends ...So she was sitting up with her legs that out, and then my other best friend and I had our heads on her like we were laying on her legs, and we were all the three of us just watching the sunset. and I just felt so at peace and so happy, and just like very in the moment and like I started crying, They're

like, 'oh, my God! Are you okay?' And I was like, 'No, it's all good. I'm healing like...' ... look at that moment I knew like everything's fine, like what had happened the years before that didn't matter like from like that moment... I was like...I know it's all gonna be fine. It's all gonna be okay. I actually have a picture of like us to laying down on her legs. She took a picture. She was like "this is so cute with the sun setting" so I every now and again, if I'm like feeling really kind of I don't know rattled, or like, just something's off. I'll like go back, and I'll look at that picture, and I'm like 'okay it like you will. There are good days like there'll be more moments like that when you are just so at peace. So, it like you're fine. It's okay, like whatever you feeling now that's a good tooth like valid. But like you're okay. It's gonna it's gonna get better.'

To reflect this **moment of relief and empowerment**, Christina shared a photo as an artifact that signifies a moment that healing and recovery from trauma is possible for her:

Image 1

Artifact shared by Christina on moments of healing from sexual trauma

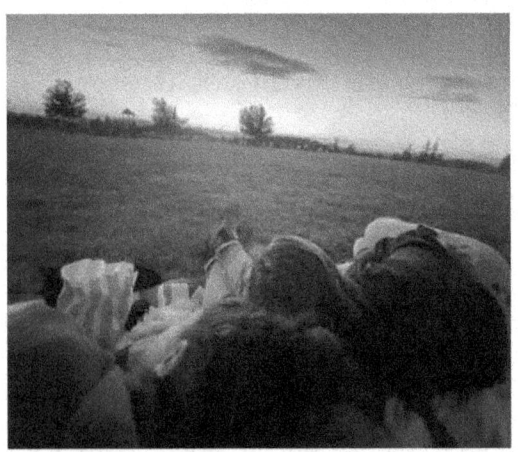

Nathan: ...um...[silence, shifting sitting position] I told you that story about how we were doing a presentation on a book that was that ...in one of my classes they were doing presentation ...before the women who were doing that presentation ... I had pulled one of them aside because I had known her personally and worked with her on another project... I had pulled her aside and said 'can you please...just experiences to the boys and men experiences...because I think it's really important' ...and at first she kind of looked at me a little skeptically like "why... where are your getting at?" and then I said "because it's really important. Because I [went] through something like this and I just wanna make sure that all people are represented" and she said "yeah, I'll see what I can do. Thank you for telling me" and that was the moment that I realized 'I think I'm saying this because I don't want other people... I don't want it to be a misconception that it doesn't happen to men or that it's something that's very rare' because I don't think it's as rare as some people might think it is.

Nichole: there's those couple weeks where it definitely my behavior was different, and then I remember making the decision not to dress myself for my aggressor (Nicole laughs) just like "You're not getting dressed for him!" Like I looked in the mirror and I was like "You're not choosing clothes for him! That's just not what you're doing. And um I wore whatever I wanted for that day..And I was able to sort of, I like I like...um ...uh sort of like having a system for myself so I had sort of staggered...easing myself back into, um, wearing my clothes. (Nichole laughs)

All the stories and experiences included in the **moments of relief and empowerment** were described by participants as tentative but positive reminders of personal growth. For some participants like Nathan, having a choice and deciding the *purpose of disclosure* and receiving positive outcomes and support from others have contributed to **moments of relief and empowerment**. Participants shared having experienced multiple encounters and moments related to personal awareness, while others were able to specifically recall moments that reminded them of their healing.

Round one emerging processes

During the first-round analysis, detailed explanation was provided by participants on the experiences after encountering sexual violence. In addition, some PROCESSES, written in capital letters here after, were identified. These PROCESSES showed the relationship within a **category** and between and among **categories**, *properties*, and dimensions. The first PROCESS was AUTHENTICITY LEADS TO POSITIVE TRAUMA RESPONSE AND MOMENTS OF RELIEF. This refers the relation of congruence and authenticity in participants sense of self and their presence within their social context with the positive experiences of responses to trauma. authentic presence was also related to experiencing **moments of relief and empowerment**. The second PROCESS was ACCEPTANCE BY OTHERS FACILITATES IDENTITY EXPLORATION AND FORMATION. Participants shared the importance of acceptance by those around them upon disclosing both identity related information and their encounter with sexual trauma. The third PROCESS that was identified during the first-round analysis was ENCOUNTERS WITH THE SYSTEM SHAPES DECISIONS OF REPORTING SEXUAL VIOLENCE. Participants discussed both their personal encounter with the police and the judicial system that contributed to their decision to not report their experience with sexual violence to the police. The last PROCESS was the PROCESSES WITHIN RESPONDING TO TRAUMA. This PROCESS focuses on participants' report on the cyclical nature of trauma response.

Authenticity leads to positive trauma response and moments of relief. Participants' *authenticity*, a *property* under **responding to trauma,** is expressed through the congruence between their *gender identity* and their identity expression and can positively facilitate the journey after sexual violence. Most participants discussed the benefits of living an authentic life as they integrate trauma into their self-image and self-worth. *Authentic* presence in the world was associated with better relationships. One participant disclosed the changes in the quality of his friendships now that his self-awareness has increased:

> **Tim Samson:** I mean one thing I will say, like I don't think I have any authentic friendships outside of my marriage until I came to [an educational setting] that includes my previous grad school experience, like because I was never able to totally be me. So, all of my acquaintances, my friendships for like based in this version of me that felt really fake, I didn't know how fake it was until... looking within and like doing all that work. But I don't think I'm not done by any search [of] the imagination. But like I'm showing up authentically every day now

Although these intentional decisions of *authenticity* have been associated with positive outcomes for participants, the becoming process has not been easy. For Sophie, the ongoing unintentional inauthenticity is shown during sexual encounters:

> **Sophie:** totally, yeah totally, especially even just in those sexual interactions like I don't feel like it .... I... it's a fully authentic experience for me. Not that I'm faking

something but that I'm not fully showing up...right? like yeah, I am like guarded I guess guarded [with soft voice] ...uhmm.... definitely distracted.

Sophie recognized the inauthentic and distracted presence during sexual encounters as a barrier to the healing journey:

> **Sophie:** I think the more detached you are from something the less of a corrective experience it can be, right? so even if I had safe sex while I was wasted ...um...you know how much am I really processing? How much is my body really processing safety while being literally interconnected with another person ..um...so I ...I imagine that if I could be, you know, the more I imagine a correlation between authenticity and healing.

Similarly, hiking was associated with being introspective and reflecting about identities. One participant talked about the realization he had about his gender identity during one of these hikes:

> **Tim Samson:** and like I was out on a hike, and I was sitting by myself, and I realized, like out here I don't feel male, like I feel ...me and I am not defined by the society's construct of what it means to have a penis. and that really was.... God, it feels good.

Participants experiences with **moments of relief and empowerment** were also related to participants' *authentic* presence in their daily life and professional work as well as in their connectedness with those around them.

> **Tim Samson:** I can look at somebody. and I can be like "It's just all about you". and I don't think I could have like that's weirdly like that disengagement self is something that I couldn't have done like that's real evidence to healing.

> **Nichole:** Umm... I also remember the first time I decided to hug a friend (short pause) again. Umm, just when we saw each other before class...Umm (pauses) yeah that didn't feel like a decision, but I was like "Oh yeah, I mean, so that, they like, the touch felt natural and safe here so I... I engaged that".

Acceptance by others facilitates identity exploration and formation. As participants explored their sexual and gender identity, they considered their **sociocultural contexts** mainly due to the fear of not being accepted were they to identify and present congruently with how they perceive themselves. Positive experience of sexual orientation exploration and formation was facilitated by the realization that their culture and identity do not have to be in conflict. The following two participants talked about this experience of realizing the intersection of culture with their identity and their experience dealing with the challenge:

> **Christina:** So, when I was kind of put forward with it [sexual orientation], I actually had to deal with it [conflict with Hispanic culture] a little bit. It almost got to the point where I felt like I had to choose myself over my culture and my family. But then, when I realized, like I actually didn't have to. I can still have my culture. I could still have part of my family.
>
> **Nichole:** I also knew that I wouldn't find a church quite as accepting and affirming, I am queer, as the one that I was at in [city] um so I just needed something else to be in that place.

Encounters with the system shapes decisions of reporting sexual violence.

Participants' racial awareness, coupled with the consistent evidence of systemic oppression against people of color as witnessed in their lives, influenced the decisions participants made following sexual violence. For instance, Nichole shared their decision to not report the sexual violence to the police.

> **Nichole:** I'm obviously brown and then other ways obviously queer too… like whoever whatever like white cowboy was going to be the one handling the case …basically, I just didn't want to be the recipient of any more evidence of the world is the way it is[laughter]
>
> **River:** in New Orleans in 2006, there was a few of us sitting outside this bar waiting for a show and three cop cars showed up, and …we were wearing dirty T-shirts and stuff, we were just traveling and they told us all [to]line up on the wall, and like searched all our pockets and the girl next to me, the cop was like reaching his hands like as far as he could in the pockets and she was like trying not to cry and he was like "what's wrong? Did your daddy touch you too much? Or did he not touch you enough?" and at that point I just wanted to like, obviously you don't punch cops, but in my head [I wanted to punch the cop]… And then he's got to me and firmly grabbed my breast, and then like search my back pockets. I had nothing.

Processes within responding to trauma. Participants shared that self-talk has contributed to developing their self-awareness. Self-awareness was related to participants' growth mindset by advancing their ability to recognize their *emotional responses* as well as to develop coping skills. Similarly, Tim Samson also describes the importance of self-awareness for positive personal growth and self-worth:

> **Tim Samson:** …and how much of the emptiness that created. Coz you could never get that void filled if you don't know what the void is.

Empathy was also related to the act of seeking forgiveness from trusted others. One participant shared that because of the connectedness he felt with women, who are mostly subjected to misogyny in society, he felt that he needed to apologize to his current partner for any past intentional or unintentional objectification of her:

> **Nathan:** and … I remember talking to my partner and asking did you ever think these things about me? did you ever think that I was abusive? or I was cruel because if I was, I'm very sorry.

Therefore, empathy following traumatic experiences allowed participants to be intentional when sharing space with others, to recognize the challenges experienced due to **sociocultural contexts** both for them and others who share underrepresented identities, and to carry the *survivor's emotional burden* of questioning and advocating for others. Naming and normalizing positively facilitated participants' journey to self-awareness, self-trust, disclosure to others and self-worth. Normalizing experiences have come from others upon intentional or unintentional disclosure of having experienced sexual violence. Sophie shared that her partners' ability to disclose about past family diagnosis and traumatic symptoms helped provide an assurance that she could be accepted by others despite the panic attacks that occurred during a sexual interaction:

> **Sophie:** he [her partner] responded by saying like "Oh my dad has PTSD and so I know what some of that looks like" and so that that helped too as a verbal processor to feel not just like tolerated but like accepted and seen and still wanted.

Overall, the PROCESSES in round-one analysis were indicative of the emerging relationships within and among **categories,** *subcategories, properties,* and dimensions that were identified during the first-round analysis. Participants authentic existence was related to positive trauma responses which latter contribute to experiences of moments of relief. Participant who had past negative encounter with the legal and judicial system explicitly stated their decision to not report their experience with sexual trauma. These preliminary PROCESSES also indicate the cyclical nature of the properties and dimensions of **responding to trauma.**

Summary of first-round interview

During the first-round interview, seven **categories** including **sociocultural contexts, identity exploration and formation, pre-trauma self and relationships, the perpetrator, disclosure, responding to trauma, and moments of relief and empowerment** were identified.

Participants shared their experiences with encountering and managing **sociocultural contexts** and situations as a member of an underrepresented group. These **sociocultural contexts** shaped participants' understanding of themselves and their multiple identities, and determined the actions they took following sexual violence. They shared that the *family culture and socialization* related to their identities, and the meaning given to sexual violence determined their ability to recognize and name sexual encounters as violence and as traumatic. In addition, the individualized and collective *survivor's encounters with the system* shaped their journey following sexual violence including determining their decision of whether or not to seek justice through the legal system. As participants encountered the system including "isms", they found themselves in a place of questioning the existing social norms that led them to carry the *survivor's emotional burden* of advocating on behalf of themselves and others.

These **sociocultural contexts** and situations were also connected with participants' experience of **identity exploration and formation**. Salient identities related to *race, sexual orientation, gender identity* and *disability* status were discussed by participants. Most participants shared the importance of social support and acceptance as they explored and formed their identities. Stigma and fear of rejection of these underrepresented identities were associated with additional layers of the challenges for participants, whereas authentic expressions of these identities were helpful in navigating trauma recovery.

Participants also shared the value of a well-formed *sense of self* prior to the sexual violence to help them externalize the blame. Under the **category** of **pre-trauma self and relationships**, participants discussed the relationships and trust they formed with the perpetrator before the sexual violence. This relationship, for some participants, led to an awareness that sexual violence could come from trusted others instead of strangers. This shift from questioning to formulating an understanding of consent has helped participants to start to name and normalize their experience. On the other hand, *trusted relationships with others* who are supportive and were able to provide a sense of belongingness were reported as beneficial to participants.

The authority, power and privilege **the perpetrator** held at the time of sexual violence were also associated with the experiences after sexual violence. Under this category, participants shared that the *perpetrator's identity* contributed to their constant caution and safety concern towards those who identify similarly. Moreover, the *perpetrator's attempt to* *contact the survivor*, especially when done without any acknowledgement of the wrongdoing, was triggering to participants.

With regard to **responding to trauma,** participants shared a variety of intersecting responses that followed the experience of sexual violence. These responses are *subcategorized* as *somatic responses, emotional responses, psychological responses,* and *behavioral responses. Somatic responses* are marked by the ongoing nature of physiological reactions as a result of the sexual violence experience. These *somatic responses* were, at times, triggered by an inability to secure physical distance from the perpetrator. Moreover, some participants specifically discussed triggers during consensual sexual encounters while others discussed the general triggering caused by encounters with the system as they navigated life after experiencing sexual violence. Participants also shared their *emotional responses* following sexual violence that were marked by an increased *emotional awareness* that helped them to process their traumatic experience. Anger and *shame and guilt* were emotions that were repeatedly discussed by participants as common emotional experiences following sexual violence.

When discussing the *psychological responses* as an experience of **responding to trauma,** participants shared the use of positive self-talk, self-worth, and self-awareness as helpful in facilitating their trauma recovery. They also shared that their process of naming, accepting, and normalizing the sexual violence experience has been helpful. Participants highlighted the importance of *authenticity* in their journey as a survivor and a minority. They also shared their *behavioral responses* to sexual violence as indicated by participants' attempts to learn more about trauma and trauma responses, seeking and attending *therapy*. In addition, *behavioral responses* included "cathartic" moments of *journaling and writing* as well as engaging in *body movements* that, at times, created spiritual connections with their body and physical environment.

Participants also shared their experience of disclosing the sexual violence experience with others. **Disclosure** constituted the *intrapersonal considerations of disclosure* by survivors in either intentionally or unintentionally sharing sexual violence with others. Intentional disclosures were related to the *purpose of disclosing* in which participants considered the *why* of disclosure before sharing their experience. Unintentional disclosures were experienced when participants had visible somatic responses that were recognized by others around them. The shift from unintentional disclosure to intentional disclosure helped participants to have a choice in disclosing. After disclosure, participants also faced the *interpersonal outcomes of disclosure.* These outcomes were marked by either support from significant others or questioning the validity of the survivors' experience. Participants shared that social support from parents, friends, romantic partners, and acquaintances had positive outcomes for trauma recovery while victim questioning was associated with negative outcomes.

Finally, participants shared the **moments of relief and empowerment** that helped them in their healing journey by reminding them of moments of healing. These **moments of relief and empowerment** are marked by positive experiences of personal growth and trauma recovery. These experiences range from specific moments that participants recall as a reminder that they are healing to collective evidence of self-growth.

During the first-round analysis, participants discussed process-oriented experiences as they shared the journey following sexual trauma. These process-oriented experiences are represented in most of the categories summarized above. For instance, under the **responding** to trauma, all of the participants' disclosures related to psychological responses were dimensions where participants shared the processes involved in their journey of healing from sexual trauma. As a result, a conceptual map representing the process of surviving sexual trauma emerged during the first-round interview, in which I created an image that represents participants' experiences and processes of surviving sexual trauma. However, not all the processes were clear during the first-round interview and some categories still remain disconnected from one another.

Through the first-round analysis, I learned a lot about participants' experiences with **sociocultural contexts, identity exploration and formation, pre-trauma self and relationships, the perpetrator, disclosure, responding to trauma,** and **moments of relief and empowerment.** Some categories such as disclosure were helpful in showing both the intrapersonal and interpersonal processes as participants navigated the recovery journey from sexual trauma. However, not all of the processes and movement within these experiences following sexual violence were clear during this round of interviews. As a result, conducting a follow up, second-round interview assisted in providing clarity to the connections between and among the **categories** identified during the first-round interview. Specifically, gaps were identified on whether or not there was a relation between **power and privilege** with the experience of process of **trauma response,** if **moments of relief** related to trauma were different or similar to **moments of relief** from systemic oppression. Since participants did not discuss the concept of time during the first-round interview, I also was interested to learn whether time has a role in their trauma response.

CHAPTER 4: SECOND-ROUND ANALYSES

In this chapter, I discuss the results of second-round analyses. I quote participant voices that support the experience of encountering sexual violence and the journey following this experience. These quotes in some cases confirm and elaborate the **categories**, *subcategories*, properties, and dimensions that were identified in the first round of analyses and in other cases are used to rename and reconceptualize the themes that were identified during the first-round analyses. As a result, newly constructed, reconceptualized, renamed and/or redefined **categories**, *subcategories*, properties, and dimensions based on the second-round analyses are also be included. PROCESSES supporting the experience following the sexual violence and later used to create the conceptual map are also discussed in this chapter.

Review of procedures

The second-round interview was conducted approximately two months after the first-round interview. I used text messages or email to invite participants to participate in the second-round interview, depending on which was used as a primary mode of communication during the first-round interview process. I asked participants to bring artwork/artifacts (such as any essays, poems, songs, pictures/images, paintings, etc.) that were authored either by themselves or others and that they felt somehow represented their journey with sexual trauma. Of the six participants, five shared the artifact in the after the second-round interview. One participant had already shared an artifact immediately after the first-round interview.

Similar to the first-round interview questions, I used semi-structured guiding questions during the second-round interview. The following semi-structured questions were designed to expand the themes and understand the processes within and between the categories identified during the first-round analyses:

1. Thank you for bringing an artifact with you today, can you tell me about it and the meaning it holds in your healing process?
2. What role has time played in your journey after sexual trauma?
3. How do you think your intersecting identities (as a queer/person of color/gender minority/disabled) relate to your responses to sexual trauma?
4. Have you experienced moments of relief from systemic oppression? If so, how are those moments of relief related to or different from your moments of relief from sexual trauma?
5. How did your perpetrator hold power in the world (e.g., as a white male)? Did their power and privilege impact your process of healing?
6. Looking back on your healing journey from where you are now, what meaning do you make of your process?
7. Is there anything we haven't talked about in your healing process that you'd like me to know about?

I also asked follow-up questions based on the disclosures made by participants. Four interviews were conducted in person and the other two on Zoom. I recorded all six interviews and used Zoom transcriptions and the Word voice dictation tool to create the first draft of the transcripts. Once the transcripts were edited and finalized, they were uploaded on NVivo version12. I then used open coding to identify new codes and emerging themes and focused coding to supplement codes that were identified. No revision was made to the research design and methods during the second-round interview and analysis.

Data analyses

I analyzed the transcripts using initial coding and focused coding. Initial coding was used when participants shared new experiences and processes that hadn't been discussed during the first-round interview. In this initial coding process, I conducted line-by-line and incident-by-incident coding. Focused coding was conducted to explain and clarify the themes identified during both rounds of the interviews. Through axial coding, I identified the connections within and among the major themes that were later named as PROCESSES, identified through the focused coding. In identifying the major themes, I used the same procedure as the first-round analyses by creating **categories,** *subcategories, properties,* and dimensions. **Categories** include experiences that were discussed by a majority of the participants, while the *subcategories, properties,* and dimensions were not necessarily discussed by a majority of the participants.

Based on the call of this study to share artwork/artifacts, all six participants shared a poem, photo, lyric, or reflective essay that they believed portrayed their experience with sexual trauma. The meaning given to these artwork/artifacts by participants represented different categories that emerged in this study. Christina shared a photo that corresponded with an internal **moment of relief** from sexual trauma. She shared that the photo was an indication that healing from the multiple sexual violence encounters was possible. Nichole shared a poem and a lyric that represented a positive relationship with their body and reiterated the importance of owning and loving their body unapologetically. River shared a reflective essay she wrote that detailed the actual sexual violence encounter and the meaning she created from this traumatic incident. She also included aspects of her healing journey that have been helpful to her such as time, effort, and the #MeToo Movement. Sophie shared a lyric of a song that reflected the frustration of encountering triggers, of finding oneself in an active state of negative somatic and emotional responses despite all the time and intentional effort exerted to heal from sexual trauma. Tim Samson shared a poem he wrote that reflected his righteous anger towards the system that enabled the repetitive sexual violence he encountered and how he continues to heal from it. Nathan shared a poem he wrote for his poetry class that detailed the events during the sexual violence and its impact in social and educational settings as well as other relationship encounters. In addition to the poem, during the second-round interview, Nathan discussed the meaning associated with a song lyric he wrote to reflect the importance of strengthening connections with significant others to continue the journey of healing. Nathan did not share the actual song lyric by the time this study was finalized. These artworks/artifacts were used to support and add to the depth and clarity of the **categories,** *subcategories, properties,* and dimensions identified in the data analyses.

Experiences of sexual trauma

Following the second-round analyses, significant changes were made to the **categories,** *subcategories, properties,* and dimensions identified during first-round analyses. Some categories remained the same and others were merged into another category. Here, I summarize all changes made during second round analyses, by **category**.

The **category** of **sociocultural contexts** was renamed **sociocultural contexts and socializations**. Then, the *subcategory* of *family culture and socialization*, originally under the **sociocultural contexts category**, was broken down into to two *subcategories*: *family culture and upbringings* and *identity socializations* under the reconceptualized **sociocultural contexts and socializations category**. Additionally, two previously identified categories were combined into this newly formulated **category** as subcategories: *identity exploration and formation*, and *pre-trauma self and relationships*. The original *subcategories* under *identity exploration and formation* are now considered as *properties: racial identity, gender identity, sexual orientation,* and *disability identity.* The definitions of the *identity exploration and formation subcategory* and its *properties* remained the same. Additional quotes identified during the second-round analyses supporting these *properties* were included in these analyses to clarify and elaborate participants' experience of minority identity. For *pre-trauma self and relationships,* the original *subcategories* are now considered *properties.* Moreover, the *property* of *relationship with the perpetrator,* under *pre-trauma self and relationships subcategory,* was renamed as *relationship with the aggressor.* The definition and supporting quotes under *relationship with the aggressor* remained the same as those in the *relationship with the perpetrator* identified during first-round analyses. Very few additional quotes were added under the *pre-trauma self and relationships* based on the results of second-round analyses because participants did not revisit this *subcategory* in detail. In summary, the newly formed **category** of **sociocultural contexts and socializations** is now supported by four *subcategories: family culture and upbringings, identity socializations, identity exploration and formation,* and *pre-trauma self-and relationships.*

After the second-round analyses, a new **category** of **power and privilege** was created. **The perpetrator,** an independent category after first-round analyses, is now named as *aggressor's power and privilege* and reconceptualized as a *subcategory* under **power and privilege.** Furthermore, the original *subcategories* under **the perpetrator** were reconceptualized and became *properties.* Following the second-round analyses, the *subcategory* of *aggressor's power and privilege* has four *properties: privileged racial and* *gender identity, physical strength, positional and social power, and intersections of minority and privileged identities of the aggress*or. An additional new *subcategory* of *survivor's power and privilege* was also created under **power and privilege** that speaks to the identity-based encounters participants had within their social and contextual system as well as the emotional burden associated with questioning, acquiring knowledge and speaking up against these social systems. This *subcategory* consists of one *property: emotional burden* and a <u>dimension of encounters with the system.</u> The *emotional burden* and <u>encounters with the system</u> were initially identified as *subcategories* under the **sociocultural contexts** during first round analyses but now are moved under the *survivor's power and privilege subcategory* as *property* and <u>dimension</u> respectively. The definition and conceptualization of <u>encounters with the system</u>, and *emotional burden* remained the same.

The **category** of responding to trauma was renamed as **trauma response** and its *subcategories* of *somatic responses, emotional responses, psychological responses,* and *behavioral responses* remained the same. Additional quotes from second-round analyses were added to expand on these subcategories. However, changes were made in the *properties* and dimensions under the *subcategories* of **trauma response**. As a result, the *property* of *distance from the perpetrator* under the *behavioral responses* was renamed as *maintaining physical boundary*. The <u>dimension</u> of <u>naming and normalizing</u> under *the psychological responses subcategory* was also renamed and reconceptualized as the PROCESS, written in capital letters here after, of RECOGNIZING SEXUAL ENCOUNTER AS VIOLENCE. A new PROCESS of INTERNALIZING BLAME TO EXTERNALIZING BLAME was also created under the *psychological responses.* TIME AND INTENTIONAL EFFORT were identified as PROCESSES that interact significantly and continuously with the trauma response following the encounter of sexual violence. Additional PROCESSES that emerged during the second-round interview were also included in this chapter.

The **category** of **disclosure** and its supporting *subcategories* and *properties* remained the same after the second round of analyses. No modifications were made.

The **category** of **moments of relief and empowerment** was renamed as **moments of relief** and then its dimension of specific moments of relief to recognition of overall personal growth was merged under the *subcategories* of *internal relief* and *external relief*.

Additional changes following the second-round analyses included reconceptualizing the SHIFT IN UNDERSTANDING OF CONSENT, renamed from shift from questioning to formulating an understanding of consent dimension under the first-round analyses *subcategory* of *family culture and socialization*. This became a PROCESS connecting sexual violence, RECOGNIZING SEXUAL ENCOUNTER AS VIOLENCE and **trauma response**. Additional PROCESSES were also created following second-round analyses that connected the **categories** and *subcategories*. Figure 5 is a visual depiction of the categories, subcategories, properties, dimensions, and processes described above.

Figure 5

The Healing Journey from Sexual Trauma

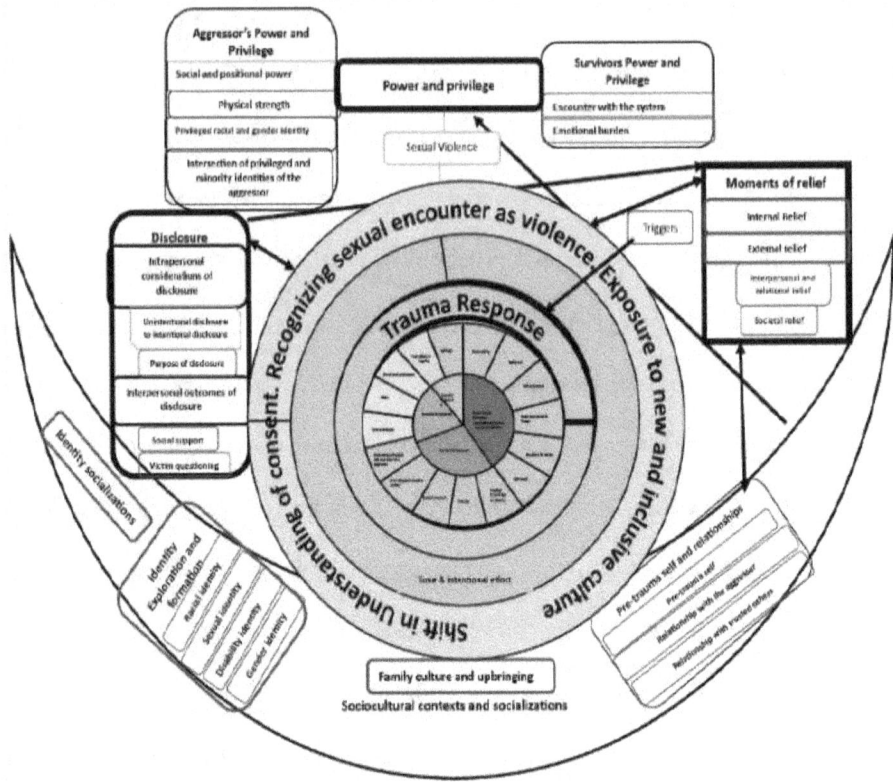

Here I will provide definitions, descriptions, and quotes from second-round interviews that supported these **categories,** *subcategories,* *properties,* dimensions, and PROCESSES. Similar to the findings of first-round analyses, the **category** of **sociocultural contexts and socialization** remained the foundation for the experience and process after encountering sexual violence.

Sociocultural contexts and socialization

This **category** was clarified and reconceptualized as family and cultural norms, stereotypes and identity socializations that shape participants' identity exploration and formation, and the development of their sense of self as they navigate social and cultural contexts both as survivors of sexual violence and as members of an underrepresented group. The **sociocultural contexts and socialization** category has four *subcategories: family culture and upbringings, identity socializations, identity exploration and formation,* and *pre-trauma self and relationships.*

Family culture and upbringings. This *subcategory* addresses the family norms and cultures that shape the actions and perspectives of participants as they form their identities and develop a sense of self. The *family culture and upbringings* played a significant role in participants' understanding of sexuality and sexual behaviors, norms of disclosure and privacy, and acceptable identities:

> **Christina:** …and coming from like a Latin, um a Latin family it (pause) you don't really talk about things. Normally, I'll go into a conversation with my family, knowing if I say something, it's gonna be family news. I'll be like 'Mom, don't say, don't tell anyone.' But in her head is "don't tell anyone that's not family." …I don't want her to talk about that [sexual violence], so I won't share that until I've healed, until I'm ready for it to be talked about. That wasn't the situation that ended up happening. She was very respectful and was like "no, I won't say anything." I didn't know that at the time before telling her …

> **Christina:** It [sexual violence] was never something that I could talk about. Already, with my family, they were like "no boyfriends until you get your PhD" like basically "stay home [and] study. That's what you need to do." We don't talk about relationships. Relationships like that's for you way down the line, and, like my parents, never talked about their relationship. They were never very affectionate in front of us. Like it's… it was just, it was a little taboo. You don't talk about it….so with that, and then combining it with like, you don't talk about your like, if something's bad, you don't really talk about it until you're ready for more, like quite a few people to know. Or you won't talk about it at all! It was a little isolating. Not feeling that support from at least my family. But again, I didn't tell them, so how would they support me? So, it was just that, like back and forth of I would want to tell them,

> **Nathan:** I was raised in two different households. My mom and dad were divorced. Um so, I had one form of parenting from my mom, and another form of parenting from my dad and they were very different. My mom was very religious, and I had no ill will towards her faith or anything. I don't. But she would often, um, she saw most sexual acts, something that need to be very private and are, it's like shameful. And I remember one thing that she used to kind of really [silence] try to teach, I guess, like

impose was that if there wasn't any feelings or some sort of… there was[not] any feelings, or intimate romance, there shouldn't be anything sexual going on

Based on participants' experiences, the *family culture and upbringing* shaped their understanding of acceptable disclosures regarding sexual behaviors and relationships as well as the norms for privacy upon disclosure. These family norms influenced the participants' decision about whether or not to disclose their sexual trauma, impacting their opportunity to obtain support in a timely manner.

Identity socializations. This *subcategory* was created out of the previous *subcategory* of *family culture and socialization* to differentiate the message participants receive from their family versus society. Based on participants' experiences, these messages of *identity socialization* were general cultural understandings of who should behave in what ways to be accepted and fit within their social surroundings. During the second-round interview, participants focused on *identity socializations* related to masculinity and femininity, and shared the cultural norms around the disclosure of negative emotions:

> **Nathan:** Yeah, I think like one of the …I remember being with my Myola, which is a grandmother in Tagalog, and my Nina, which is godmother, or it can be aunt too, I was with them, and they were talking about how …they were asking me if I had a bunch of side girls on the side. And they were like…because, you know, that's how all the men in our family are. They all do. They always have it. It's just how they are, and like they were laughing about it, thinking it was funny. And I remember thinking that I didn't know that was funny, because I also came from like my mom; my mom raised me. All that was like wrong. Having that kind of thing is not culturally acceptable, because my mom's, you know, very religious, and she's very so [silence] When I was initially processing the events [sexual violence] that transpired when I was processing my assault, there was an aspect to it that I often wondered if, like, should there be something, should I look at it in a more positive way, because the men in my family probably would, but it didn't feel positive… if I were to talk to my actual dad about this, my dad, he probably "is [it] not a good thing? You wow, kiddo! You have a lot of girlfriends that's good."
>
> **River:** …and I realized that Southern culture is very messed up in a lot of ways [laughter], and for a lot of part, especially women in the South are taught to just shut up and take it for a lack of better [word]. You know, it's like "no, you're not supposed

to make waves. You're not supposed to, you know, make people uncomfortable." And I'm just like, 'why?' [laughter]

Tim Samson: I grew up in a rural town in Northern [West] and it was, you know, I think we had one person of color in my entire high school, like it was very much like it was a homogeneous culture, like everybody, went to the same church [laughter] It was like we all like. It was very clearly defined, and there were a couple of kids who were like pretty obviously queer in some way. And they were bullied, you know. So it was like you, either, like. Don't do that like [laughter] You just all in line and be like everybody else, and I was decent enough at that, because I was good at sports.

Christina: ...but I felt like cult-, even culturally, like you don't really talk about negative emotions. Talk about all the positive ones all you like, that's fine. But negative emotions. That's your problem. That's for you to process for you to deal with like.

Moreover, one participant shared the intersection of these *identity socializations* to their experience with sexual trauma:

Nichole: I wonder (pauses) if sexual trauma, what if? (long pause) Like I wonder if, if actually (pause) I relate to the events as something more like racial trauma or homophobia or transphobia? (pause) (nervous laughter) so (pause) yeah, maybe you can figure that out on your study for me (laughs). Yeah, because it did, I didn't experience it as a sexual... being, I experienced as a racialized one and a gendered one. And so those things are definitely system, more like systemic.

These *identity socialization* messages were also repeated in collective settings where participants witnessed the impact of undermining the voices of survivors who identify as men. Nathan's artifact, a poem he wrote representing the sexual violence experience, specifically states these societal assumptions on masculinity and its impact on him as a survivor of sexual trauma:

> *One lecture, my professor speaks on the concept of toxic masculinity.*
> *Someone raises their hand, claims that toxic masculinity is innate to men, that*
> *men suppress their emotions due to social constructs. I hear Hailey*
> [aggressor] *again. How she said it* [sexual violence] *can't happen to men.*

Participants described the conflicting messages about sexual behaviors surrounding their experience with sexual trauma, and these limited their disclosure once the trauma occurred. The culture around not sharing negative emotions had delayed participants' disclosure of sexual violence that in turn led participants to process the trauma without the support of their significant others. General cultural and socialization messages towards femininity, or forcing those who identify in the femininity spectrum to "be nice," also influenced the participants' ability to speak up and advocate for themselves and others.

Identity exploration and formation. The third *subcategory* under the **sociocultural contexts and socializations** was a theme that emerged based on the first-round analyses. This *subcategory* was confirmed and further elaborated by participants during the second-round interview. During the first-round interview, participants talked about the role of *racial identity, sexual orientation, gender identity,* and *disability identity* exploration and formations as prominent parts of their journey as they encountered the sociocultural and contextual factors while navigating their experience after sexual violence.

In the second-round analyses, one participant revisited his racial identity development as a Caucasian, and his experience of recognizing and acknowledging the perceived power and privilege associated with his identity. Specifically, Tim Samson clarified and elaborated the role "white privilege" and "white guilt" played as he experienced the sexual violence 15 years ago:

> **Tim Samson:** ...and then subsequently, how much like that [sexual violence] was right around the time where I started to be like words like white privilege. And things like that we're starting to trickle into, this is like mid 2000, so like, I'm just sort of awakening to like social movements, you know, that are outside of my lived experience. And I'm starting to think 'Oh, maybe' I'm like 'there's a problem socially here' and 'oh, man, I'm the villain!' And so, there's [laughter], you know, stages of racial identity that, you know, come into play. And I was [at] a very early stage at that point. And so, the immediate reaction there was to sort of just try to be likeable [laughter]. And weirdly that kept making me want to center myself with my likable attributes like 'I'm charming. I'm fun. I can do lots of stuff at parties like I can like I could be entertaining' and sort of forming an identity around being charming and fun and talented ironically... and talented for things that I never like chose.

> **Tim Samson:** I was just like sort of shoved into those spaces. So again, that lack of control thing but the upshot of all that sort of avoidance of admitting that bad things could have happened to somebody who has as much privilege as me was that I never even acknowledged it.

Tim Samson further elaborates on the role of "white guilt," especially early during his racial identity development, and how it contributed to his silence and inability to name the events as sexual violence and trauma. He explained the denial of traumatic experiences intersecting with early white identity development and a heightened level of white guilt:

> **Tim Samson:** …that [social justice movements on oppression and privilege] early on was also happening on the side…I think the really unfortunate sort of first response that a lot of people have when they occupy a position of privilege is to feel guilt and then and go and like, so they're operating in those places like, 'I'm so sorry. I'm sorry that everything about me is the worst, and I am just going to pretend like I could never have [any problems].' I think, one of the manifestations that comes up a lot for male presenting people is that, well, especially for well-meaning at least, like 'well, I am the problem. Therefore, I can't have problems.' That's how that's how it manifested.

Tim Samson explained that the thought of naming and recognizing the sexual violence was halted by the white guilt and led to the thought that he was not supposed to have "problems" because "I am the problem." As a result, the naming and recognition of inappropriate and unwanted sexual advances were delayed:

> **Tim Samson:** … and then even to acknowledge that it has, that it had [the sexual violence occurred onto him]. That happened, that it was a bad thing like [it] can't be a bad thing because I'm not allowed to feel bad things because so many other people have it so much worse than me, you know, and this becomes the logic like, 'I'm clearly fine. I'm not, you know. Nobody physically hurt me' like 'I have a roof over my head. I have all of these privileges. This must not be a bad thing.' and I think I mean, that's a… it's [silence] it's a very perverse way of trying to reckon with white guilt, I think.

Moreover, Tim Samson's poem, the artwork/artifact submitted as an indicator of his journey with sexual trauma, points to this intersection of white privilege and recognition of trauma:

> *So I didn't even know I was hurting. Didn't know. Because I'm*
> *Successful*

White
Privileged
Not a problem
It's all my fault anyway.
There's no space for me to be traumatized because I MADE SURE OF IT.

On the privileges related to *racial identity*, Nathan talked about his mixed race and the associated **power and privilege** intersections. In this case, Nathan reported that the privilege of having mixed white race identities helped him to learn the white culture and integrate himself into the dominant culture, although he admits that he may not be granted the full "white privilege' that comes with having a full white *racial identity*:

> **Nathan:** People are always very cautious to address any of my racial identity which allows me to talk about myself and actually be like 'Oh, yeah, hey, I'm Asian', and I think it's great, and I love being Asian and I didn't always like being as a kid, but these days I do, because being Asian makes me a distinct individual with unique traits and a diverse cultural background, all of like all these different aspects like, I can be an American, and I can also go and join my family, my family on my dad's side, and like dance with all my flawless old lady friends, you know, like in Asian cultures like old ladies love to dance [smile].

> **Nathan:** And I'm also glad that I also have this white side too, because then I can also be a part of like most things, everyone else is like all the more Americanized and white people that, I don't want to sound racist, but you know,....there is a privilege component in that, um, I'm not entirely sure if I'd say that privilege component helps all that much in in terms of having, like all of a white privilege, but I do think that there is a privilege of knowing how to live with whites, if that makes sense....

He also added the views of his family and relatives on his Asian side, explaining how he is considered the "white boy" when describing the emotional burden of not fitting in with the culture of the underrepresented because of his half white *racial identity:*

> **Nathan:** in my Asian culture, when you reemerge back in there, you're always seen as still half white like you're half white, I know my cousins and even some of my Nia and Niongs and even some of my many on the they would...claim this is a white boy which it means like you're half white, through the half white boy, so it it's interesting.

For participants of color, one participant particularly, the exploration and formation of *racial identity* was intertwined with their immigrant status and culture. Nichole spoke about their process of recognizing the emotional burden associated with these identities and highlighted the moments of owning one's own identities:

> **Nichole:** it [the poem] was more about like this sort of fear that things happen to me because I'm in a brown body. Or that, like my having a brown body means that I can't have the same joys and connections as other people. But that's just not the case, so that the poem is really about like, um, (pause) I don't have to do anything to be a daughter. I am one. I don't have to do anything to be a granddaughter to my grandmother. I am one.

Nichole submitted a poem by Kalani Padilla to express their journey following the sexual violence encounter, indicating the self-reconciliation process of owning one's identity and body as well as its social role despite the societal expectation of what it means to be a person of color. This poem was written around the time of the sexual violence:

Image 2

A poem submitted by Nichole to reflect their journey after their sexual violence encounter

tadasana

by Kalani Padilla

immigrant girl mix-matches liquids in the pot, stirs, serves.
                    mistakes the mirin for the rice vinegar.
wonders if the costco on the clark fork sells oxtail. Immigrant girl
                                    makes new ears for hearing
            lullabies, even those
                    that are not sung between these mountains.[2]
immigrant girl answers "I don't
        know"
to questions about grandmother.[1]
                gets older each time.
                        immigrant girl burrows   a passage
from unhome to unhome everyday and on the way to school becomes herself   a passage.

                                    wonders
earnestly why the "freshest off the boat" would be the most undesirable.

                            smells her armpits shaves her
legs sharpens her tongue splits herself up Chicago style imagines her intended audience
carefully on either side of a horizontal line.

                    immigrant scholar is taught "defense" as an interface of
discourse between equals, then graduates
            1. immigrant scholar is accused (yes, mostly from within) of
forgetting something she was not taught.
                    immigrant child imagines wrapping Ilocano around
christmas gifts the way grandmother wraps her arm around her little sister's arm.
                                    2. recalls being a
                        child
in the Aloha Stadium parking lot during Swap Meet all alive alive alive with Ilocano.

                                Comprehends
                    that Filipino
        is not rhetoric.

    not
        passage or place.

                    granddaughter is   just you
                                    standing there.

Similarly, Nathan also shared his journey of owning his *racial identity* and shining a positive light on his mixed race:

> **Nathan:** especially as more interracial relationships are becoming more and more prominent, I have sort of a view, my Asian ethnicity, my Asian American nature as a positive thing, as something that I think that I should own, and I should be very confident especially as of as of lately.

Participants also discussed the interconnectedness of their process of forming *gender identity* and their experience and process of meaning-making following sexual violence. Tim Samson, for instance, shared the following:

> **Tim Samson:** I also think that it [the sexual violence encounters] gave me a space to explore my gender that felt really good, yeah, actually, the first time that I thought ...I think part of what felt good about leaning into and maybe getting some of these experiences that were bad was that I could be more feminine, and that was like celebrated like that for "how good!" But the "oh, but you must be gay." ... 'Nope. just the gay of straight guy.' I you know I'm so glad I've learned the term gender expansive [laughter].

To summarize, during the second round, *identity exploration and formation* was discussed as participants differentiated the power and privilege associated with *racial identity* and the experience of processing sexual violence alongside recognizing white privilege. Participants also discussed the emotional burden associated with cultural expectations and socializations related to having a mixed-race identity. Owning these privileged and nonprivileged identities and recognizing the power and privileges associated with them has been empowering for participants. The participants also talked about the intersection of early stages of *racial identity* development with *gender identity* exploration and sexual violence.

Pre-trauma self and relationships. This theme was a category on its own during the first-round analyses but was reconceptualized as a subcategory under the **sociocultural contexts and socializations** following the second-round analyses. This *subcategory* has three properties: *pre-trauma sense of self, relationship with the aggressor* and *relationship with* *trusted others*. Some participants shared the role of their *pre-trauma sense of self* as they experienced sexual violence and explored its meaning afterwards. For instance, in highlighting the sense of self he had prior to entering the entertainment world, part of Tim Samson's poem, the artwork he shared to show the experience and process of healing from sexual trauma, reads:

> *It's a funny thing*
> *Self-awareness – trying to de-center, always*
> *Finding a way back*
> *To the middle of your conversation about yourself: "oh hello, have you heard about me?"*
> *"Have you heard about the funny thing that makes me charming?"*
> *"Have you heard about the used-to-bes that make me inspirational?"*
> *"Have you heard about the party tricks that make me entertaining?"*
>
> ...
>
> *"Have you heard how I'm a terrified little boy who never learned how to feel vulnerable and centering myself in your space helps me feel like I must matter. Somehow."*
> *Record scratch or whatever.*
> *I often think about how many scared little boys there are in big scary bodies.*
> *Maybe I'm lucky that my body isn't scary.*
> *My body is...*
> *...not mine?*
> *It's America, baby, be sexy, get those abs*
> *An actual line I read on a gym ad: "If you want to get SHREDDED you gotta ROCK THE INSANITY!"*
> *As if that means something.*
> *I feel my eyes start to roll when I think of pithy sayings like "the curse of the gifted child" or "prisoner of talent". It's the same with "my body was so conventionally attractive that people paid me tens of thousands of dollars to parade it around onstage".*
> *But my path kept getting paved ahead of me by professors, casting directors, horny producers.*
> *"you can sing, you need to sing"*
> *"You can act, you need to act"*
> *"You look good with your shirt off, take it off"*
> *My well-being – sense of self – sense of autonomy*
> *My body.*
> *Not mine.*

When reflecting on this artwork during the interview, Tim Samson stated the anger he feels because his sense of self was controlled and guided by those around him:

> Tim Samson: I got angry. I was writing it [the poem] and it's something that we talked before I don't feel anger. I don't feel mad. But then, sort of like letting my memory sort of walk back there, I found myself being like that time 'I was just so out of control of my own anything' like that I was just desperate to work, you know, so like I would do anything for work, and you know I wasn't in control of my own body, and people were telling me like "this is how your voice has to sound like" and it's all sort of wrapped in this odd framework of "you're lucky to be here" and so like you just sort of jump through the hoops, and you don't really question it.

Similarly, River shared her artifact in an essay that described the events leading up to the sexual violence in relation to her pre-trauma sense of self and disability identity:

> *This was at the same time that I was misdiagnosed with bipolar. (The correct diagnosis, years later would be autism. Along with ADHD, but the ADHD I was properly diagnosed with at age 4, in 1991.) I was misdiagnosed with bipolar and put on the drug 'Abilify,' around age 14 or 15. It numbed me to a point where I simply didn't give a shit about anything, and not in a good way. Like a 4-year fever dream. I didn't question anything, I didn't even ask what drugs I was handed. Looking back, it's absolutely terrifying what it did to me, and I'm lucky to be here.*

In addition, River detailed her *relationship with the aggressor* prior to the sexual trauma. The following statement was included in her essay representing her journey of surviving sexual trauma:

> *Steven was always a bully, but because he was the kind of person that also got bullied, he somehow got away with it. I tolerated him because my friends liked him. When I was in high school, he somehow became best friends with my boyfriend and was always trying to turn Andrew against me. He had a car before my other friends, so we rode with him. Sometimes he would "joke" that he would only give me a ride if I made out with his girlfriend in front of him. Lucky for me (and her) she was a great friend, good kisser, and queer. One of those adolescent friendships that you're pretty much only in because of proximity and convenience. (Him, not her.)*

In his poem Nathan also included the relationship he had with his aggressor prior to the sexual violence encounter:

> *It started with Hailey, I hung out with her because I was lonely, lost, losing myself.*
> *I needed a friend, so she drove me out into the mountains, parking in the middle of nowhere as snowflakes gathered on her windshield, our breaths fogging the glass*

> *Hailey told me about what he did to her, how she never wanted it and no one*
> *believed her.*
> *She said how I was lucky because that sort of thing can't happen to boys.*
> *She described her turmoil, each word making my hands ball into trembling*
> *fists....*

Furthermore, Nathan explained in his poem how he did not have a choice or the opportunity to make a decision about continuing a *relationship with the aggressor* following the sexual violence:

> *...The drive back was quiet. I told her I wanted to remain friends, thinking*
> *that maybe it was my fault, that I had sent out the*
> *wrong signals, said the wrong thing, made her confused so I had to clarify.*
> *She dropped me off, sped out of my driveway, and blocked me so there was no*
> *chance of us ever speaking again...*

Overall, the **sociocultural contexts and socialization** have been foundational as participants formulate their perspectives about sexual encounters as well as explore their identities. The *family culture and upbringings* focused on participants' experiences with the family norms that influenced their understating of sexual behaviors and disclosure and privacy. *Identity socializations* were about the generalized messages of sexual behaviors, masculinity and femininity that influenced their identity development. Moreover, participants discussed the intersection of racial identity development with gender identity development contributed to their inability to name and recognize unwanted sexual advances as violence. Participants did not revisit the *pre-trauma self-and relationships* during the second-round interview.

Power and privilege

The **category** of **power and privilege** emerged after the second-round analyses, and refers to the power and privilege associated with the different and multiple identities of both participants and aggressors that impacted participants' experience of sexual violence and trauma. Two *subcategories* were identified under this **category**: *aggressor's power and privilege* and *survivor's power and privilege.*

Aggressor's power and privilege. This *subcategory* refers to the power and privilege the aggressor holds in the world in relation to their gender, race, physical strength, and position in their workplace and social circle. It also consists of the intersection of the aggressor's oppressed and privileged identities as understood by the survivors. With the exception of one sexual violence encounter reported by one participant, most of these incidents involved the aggressor having a higher power or a privileged identity compared to the survivor. In this one incident that did not involve the aggressors' power and privilege, the participant described the event as her own inability to "not stand up for myself":

> **Christina:** with that one I feel like with her. I ended up giving her more power. Of just myself not standing up as much. I don't, really. I don't really think that the second one was a power struggle, but more of just of a situation that I didn't know what to do. and instead of you know, fight or flight I freeze to the combo of I don't really know what to do in the situation, and then freaking out and just like freezing. So, I don't think the second one was very much a power one.

One participant was also unsure of the power and privilege associated with her aggressor's identity, citing her inability to differentiate the role that the aggressor's power plays in her journey following sexual violence versus a combination of secondary trauma and other traumatic experiences she endured when she was a child:

> **Sophie:** … but what's interesting is that long- even before then, that incident, I've had a lot of reactivity, um, to sexual things that makes me unsure of what my younger childhood experience-(long audio cut out)…I also experienced or just taking on a lot of secondary trauma from working with clients and not knowing how to, um, you know, hold boundaries for with myself, for that, or heal from that. And so, it's not totally clear to me who my perpetrator is. And so, it's a little tricky for me to be able to specifically identify the powers that that population held. aside from that (long audio cut off)

Despite these exceptions, participants consistently discussed the **power and privilege** their aggressor held at the time of the sexual violence. The *subcategory* of *aggressor's power and privilege* is supported by four *properties: physical strength, privileged racial and gender identity, positional and social power,* and *intersections of minority and privileged identities of the aggressor.* Below is a description of these *properties* and supporting statements based on participants' experiences.

Physical strength. This *property* refers to participants' perception that their aggressor has more physical strength compared to them. The *physical strength* of the aggressor has contributed to participants' inability to fight back during the sexual violence and/or created fear for their safety during and/or after the sexual violence. Christina, who encountered sexual violence from three aggressors on three different occasions, explained the role that the physical strength of her aggressors had on her inability to defend herself. Specifically, physical strength was a significant factor when the aggressor was male or male-identifying:

> **Christina:** He [the aggressor] was also a ROTC person. So, he had that physical advantage, and I was asleep when it all started. So, he had the power, because I was unconscious, of a straight white man. I had... I was asleep on a bed thinking I was safe. And that just wasn't that- that wasn't the case.... I was actually like trying to like use my body to get away, so high five on that one [self] (Laughs) But it, it was. Yeah, the power, like, just having that physical strength of actually like pushing away and realizing like, 'I'm not moving.' Yeah 'this is, this is it. I'm not moving.' That definitely hit. And it was it was. It was very different to the other two.

Christina reported a similar fear for safety towards an aggressor who was identifying as female. She stated the change in her views of physical strength and muscle following sexual encounters that felt violating to her:

> **Christina:** ...part of it was physical size. She's taller, stronger than me, so I felt honestly a little bit intimidated by that especially afterwards [sexual violence]. At first, I'm like, (in a cheery voice) 'Oh, she's taller than me!' and then I was like, (in a matter-of-fact voice) 'No, she's taller than me.' She... that means like... other than the

height they got a little bit more muscle, probably. So, normally with tall you go stronger.

Nichole also expressed safety fears they felt during the sexual violence due to the "aggressive" presence of their aggressor prior to the sexual encounter:

> **Nichole:** he's very aggressive, sort of volatile presence. So, I think he liked to be unpredictable. It's also, really, just like strong, like physically very strong. He was not expecting me to be as strong as I was, but he definitely could have harmed me had he known.

This physical strength imbalance as the aggressor attempted to engage in a sexual encounter with the survivor was also reported by Sophie:

> **Sophie:** ... there's one particular incident that I can think of where I, um (pause) was that I remember having, like my first (pause) like panic attack. But that was with someone who was like a friend, and who is drunk and stronger than me, who wanted to have sex, and then I, and like we almost did. But I was able to convey to him enough that I didn't want to do that, and so we stopped.

In general, the *physical strength* of the aggressor is associated with fear for the safety of the participants and contributed to the inability to defend themselves against sexual violence.

Privileged racial and gender identity. This *property* was created following the second-round analyses under the *subcategory* of *aggressor's power and privilege*. The *privileged racial and gender identity* refers to the power and privilege associated with the aggressors' gender identity and racial identity; participants discussed the intersections of the privileged status of their aggressor due to the aggressor's gender and race:

> **River:** well, he is a white dude so there's that um.... his parents give him everything he ever wanted. So, there's that.

> **Nichole:** Yeah. Well, honestly, like no one that I talked to assumed it was anyone but a white man. (laughs) So actually, it felt like, super. I didn't have to explain anything. (pauses) and I had a friend, actually, who was like, 'was it a white dude?" And it was like, and that was just so funny (laughs). It was funny to hear her say that, because, of course, it was. Hmm, first of all, there are no brown men around (laughs) um (pauses)

that's weird, too (pause). But yeah. So, I think that, like his identity made it very simple to explain, actually.

Nichole: Yeah. Yep. It feels almost too obvious [power he has due to race and gender identity] to say. Yeah. It was so weird. (pauses) What is the obvious part? (pauses) Don't know. I just feel like it's in the receipts. I do remember (pause) like, in other interactions with him, when I would try to have any sort of civil discourse, like he had not learned how to do that. Like I would try to explain something very care- like respectfully and he would just lash out without any sort of response to what I said. He just sort of felt attacked, I think, (pause) most people have experienced, like negative experiences like that with that demographic, anyway. Yeah.

In both River's and Nichole's experiences, there was a perception that white males seemed to have a predefined privileged identity that made it easier to communicate with others without necessarily having to explain due to the power that they hold in the world.

On the other hand, Nathan, whose aggressor was a white woman, explains the power and privilege associated with the aggressor's race and as well as her gender, especially when it comes to believability when disclosing sexual violence to others:

Nathan: Yeah, because male sexual [assault] is already not taken nearly as seriously as female sexual assault. And at the same time, I think that [silence] I think that ethnic people are often considered scary to most white people. I mean, we we can talk about like yellow peril or like how white women being raped was often the thing of like the cause for a lot of lynching, you know, like these types of things happen. So, I think that just being a white woman who can kind of...she has a certain value, social value, and it's different than ethnic women. And please forgive me if that's ignorant because I could be completely wrong.

The hesitance in Nathan's statement regarding the power the perpetrator holds in the world was also indicated in Sophie's description of the power of a white male aggressor:

Sophie: yeah, well. This is where it gets a little tricky for me because there's one particular incident that I can think of where I, um (pause) was that I remember having, like my first (pause) like panic attack. But that was with someone who was like a friend, and who is drunk and stronger than me, who wanted to have sex, and then I, and like we almost did. But I was able to convey to him enough that I didn't want to do that, and so we stopped. Umm, and so, but I was really, really, I remember to be really scared in that moment, until he stopped. And that was a white man. So there's that. But what's interesting is that long- even before then, that incident, I've had a lot of reactivity, um, to sexual things that makes me unsure of what my younger childhood experience-(long audio cut out)

When explaining the power associated with identifying with being white, Christina shared that her woman aggressor's white racial identity did not factor into the sexual violence experience and what followed:

> **Christina:** I guess. I never felt that she used her race as a power tool, but with that I think it's because I am very set, and being a proud Latin person, proud Mexican. So, I don't let a lot of that waiver for me. I've had partners who are like you need to basically stop being so ethnic of like stop celebrating your culture so much. And I'm like 'no!' turn on Mariachi music and dance away. So, what like, yeah, that's not going to happen. I'm proud of who I am. so I'm going to stick with that. So, I feel, in that route it was, I was okay.

The intersection of **power and privilege** associated with both the aggressor's gender and race were described by participants, especially participants of color, as having a significant role in how they processed the sexual violence. At the same time, participants Nathan and Sophie seemed hesitant to conclude with full certainty that the white race and gender identity of their aggressors contributed to their encounter with sexual violence.

Positional and social power. This *property* was created under the *aggressor's power and privilege subcategory* after the second-round analyses and refers to the *positional and social power* the aggressor held at the time of the sexual violence. The *positional and social power* refers to the aggressor's power at a workplace and/or in social relations involving the survivor. Participants described their fear of the informational, social, and positional power their aggressor held that contributed to participants' silence and/or perceived accountability for engaging in the sexual encounter. For instance, Christina reported her hesitance around fully rejecting her woman aggressor because of the fear that her parents would find out she is in a same sex relationship before coming out to them:

> **Christina:** …I was still closeted to my family, still hadn't told them at that time. And even though I knew there was like she [the first aggressor] had no contact information for my family. I also know that girls are good at finding information. So, I had a little bit of that feeling of like she could tell my family. She could just out me, and that could be dangerous for me.

Similarly, Christina's third aggressor had informational power that could jeopardize her employment giving him more social and positional power at the workplace:

> **Christina:** He was a co-worker. We were RAs together, and so R- we are RAs during Covid. So, he had the power of basically being able to get me fired by reporting that I was underage drinking [and] reporting that I had broken Covid rules by being in other people's rooms. With those two my job would have already been out the door… So, a lot of that power came because he [the aggressor] could just tell on me.

Speaking to the *positional and social power* of their aggressor, participants also highlighted differences in age, financial power and their aggressor's access to materials (including mood-altering substances) that factored into the sexual violence encounter.

> **Christina:** My first, I guess trauma, my partner lived in [small town], went to school up in [College town], and I didn't have a car, and I lived in the dorms, and she lived off campus, had her own car. She was older than me. She was like a junior in college when I was a freshman. So already with that. She was older than me. She had a car and could drive to see me. Um, so it was more of a, I guess a relationship where I was meeting her needs and when she wanted to come down to see me then I can make time…So, I think the combination of being older having, like basically the ability to tram- like to come to see me, and almost feeling like obligated of when she [aggressor] wanted to because she was making that trip. I had to see her.

> **River:** and he's you know, high schoolers, we like trying different drugs, and for whatever reason he had access to a lot of them. So, he would show up at the party with the back of whatever, and so everyone would want to be his friend because he'd be along with free drugs and like, so there was like that. And my, he always looked older than us that. So, he never got carded for anything, so he was like able to like, buy the booze, and like he like knew people that worked at liquor store. So, he had all these weird ins. And it's like, you know, when you're in high school, we just on the like party on the weekends. It's like, well, you're gonna hang out to people like him whatever.

Moreover, participants discussed the social power their aggressor held at the time of the sexual violence. Having this social power meant that participants were fearful of losing the close social network they had or of not being able to belong to their immediate social network if they were to speak up against their aggressor:

> **River:** I don't want to sit at home by myself. So, I guess I'll go to this party with this asshole...cause it was like that was like, only I would get to hang up [with] my friends things for free. And you know it's like all these social pressures. And it's like, now I'm just realizing now that was just like his like key to manipulate everyone around them.

> **Sophie:** I um (pause) was that I remember having, like my first (pause) like panic attack. But that was with someone who was like a friend, and who is drunk and stronger than me, who wanted to have sex, and then I, and like we almost did. But I was able to convey to him enough that I didn't want to do that, and so we stopped.

> **Tim Samson:** It was like so two of the big ones: one of the guys was the [person of power]. So, it was a high [financial and positional power], so like already, like he's risen to a very competitive marketplace to get to like a you know, a [head of a professional work], and that's that carries a pretty in the [previous profession] world. It carries a big degree of status, and you know, of course, me operating the lens of patriarchy like oh, status!

> **Tim Samson:** and he's beloved, and he's a sweetheart, and everybody likes him, and he's doing a great job in the [profession] and like. And he just starts focusing on me and like flirting with me and like it's flattering like and I'm like 'don't know where this is going.' Like he's I've been in it long enough to know like he's eventually try to like make a move on me but I'm playing the game... this is actually the only time I ever said like 'that went too far' like, you know, grab my grab my penis, and it was like, my, that's 'you need to stop' and ...he stopped interacting with me at all, and it became very uncomfortable. And ah [voice shaking] ...

Nathan on the other hand shared that he felt manipulated by his aggressor prior to the sexual violence, and that led him to be more empathic and trusting of her. Here is his description:

> **Nathan:** One of the things that she told me about was that, she said that she was sexually assaulted before, which is why, it was very interesting that this [his sexual violence encounter] occurred like in succession. She said that she was sexually assaulted before, and that no one believed her, and I felt so bad because hearing someone confide that in you like it's very intimate and I didn't really know how to respond. And then the entire incident just unfolded, and I was kind of thinking, like you know. I thought about a lot since, and I wonder [silence] I've often wondered. And I don't, I don't want, I don't want to be seen as like misogynistic for thinking this, but I often wonder if she uses that as a means to gain someone's if it's like it was a, it was a trick like it was like "hey, your guards [are] down and tell you about this, and then boom! I'm gonna do this to you." And then I think that if I were to have said anything to anyone as both someone who is ethnic and someone who is male. They wouldn't

believe me over someone who was white and someone who was a woman. And in that sense, there's kind of a power difference.

Under the *positional and social power*, participants discussed the power that their aggressor held by having informational power that could cause them harm, having social power amongst the social group they share with the aggressor, having supervisory power at a workplace, and having relational power over them. This impacted the participants' ability to say "no" while the sexual violence was happening, and/or decisions following the sexual violence encounter.

Intersections of minority and privileged identities of the aggressor. This *property* refers to the intersection of privileged and oppressed power in relation to the aggressors' identities. When discussing the **aggressor's power and privilege,** participants also discussed the intersection of the privileged and less privileged identities that their aggressor(s) held at the time of the sexual violence. These intersections of the aggressors' identities have influenced the meaning participants make of their experience. For instance, Nathan explained the "empathy and sympathy" he feels for women survivors of sexual trauma when discussing his emphasis on educating himself about women suffering despite the fact that his aggressor was a woman herself:

> **Nathan:** um it's very disheartening [emphasis on women survivors] but I understand, because and I, as someone who has experienced this [sexual violence], I feel sympathy and empathy towards women. So, I understand that women in general tend to have a hard, harder, and more difficult time regarding these things. So that's why we put more emphasis on them. And by using certain wording, we could potentially promote misogyny which undermines feminine struggles.

Similarly, Tim Samson explained the intersections of his aggressors' identities having an influence on the meaning he created for his process after naming the experience as sexual violence. That his aggressors held less privileged identities in the world (as gay men), despite higher professional status at their workplace, facilitated "forgiveness" for Tim Samson:

> **Tim Samson:** This is where I feel a lot of grace and a lot of forgiveness, because a lot of these guys [aggressors] like didn't hold much power in the world, because they were very, obviously, the gay men. For the most part, we might say very obviously, feminine men, and, where I can sort of code switch away from that, these guys couldn't like it was just like so baked into how they expressed themselves. And in the this isn't like the like, I said in the early [years] where like, you know, gay marriage hadn't been legalized yet, and so like their spaces, like the space where you can be non-heterosexual were very specific and I think the clichés are like "theater for boys and softball for girls"...These are the spaces where you know you're a gay man That's a safe space for you..... You go to the [previous profession]. So, these worlds become like sequestered, and within that world [the aggressors] have tons of power. So, me, entering into [previous profession] without any sense of how that power was structured, it was...I think that's how I sort of got in trouble... so two of the big ones, one of the guys was the [a person in power]. So, it was a high paid professional [in the previous profession], so like already, like he's risen to a very competitive marketplace to get to like a, you know, a [had professional and positional power], and that's that carries a pretty [high power] in the [previous profession] world. It carries a big degree of status, and you know, of course, me operating the lens of patriarchy like 'oh, status!'

Tim Samson also discussed his perception that the culture in the entertainment industry promotes blurred sexual boundaries and led his aggressors to make the unwanted sexual advances towards him:

> **Tim Samson:** ...I think that he [the aggressor] probably let that power go to his head and I think he's walked enough in those spaces where he just sort of rose to the top and wasn't really keeping himself accountable. And I was a guy who...he probably had that experience with so many other times, you know, you're in a position of power and social power and you have these sort of like less powerful people who are probably, who look and act like me [who] probably do want to have sex with you, right? And I was, you know, just kind of an oddball in that way, or like my sexual orientation wasn't his. ... um even that being said, I'm hearing the absurdity of it, you know, just because [of] my sexual orientation, [it] doesn't mean that I want to have sex with anybody who is the same orientation. But that sort of was the expectation of that culture. But there's a lot of just promiscuity.

Other situations in which the aggressors held less power include financial status, history of substance use, and being bullied at a young age:

Nichole: (pause)yeah, (pause) I don't- I feel like I, I also don't know enough about him personally to make those kinds of assumptions, maybe. It's obvious that he is a white dude. But I, I think he grew up in poverty, and so has a lot of anger. Um, that he wields freely (pause) is an alcoholic. I don't know if there any of these answers the question really, I'm just sort of trying to take stock of what I know and what that has to do with power (long pause).

River: Well, he is a white dude so there's that um...his parents give him everything he ever wanted so, there's that, and I think he saw himself as some sort of victim also, because he kind of got made fun of in middle school, because, like I don't know, he listened to like goth music, and but I had known him since middle school, and he was always something I didn't really like but he was someone that was in my circle of friends, and he was in the same grade as us but his birthday was in September so he got his license before most of my friends so we would get rides from him and stuff like that.

Reflecting through the essay she wrote as an artifact representing her journey following the sexual violence encounter, River noted the intersections of the privileged identities of her aggressor with his experience of bullying:

> *I'm sure there are a million reasons why Steven is the way he is, but honestly, I don't care. It doesn't matter because I refuse to try to justify the acts of a rapist. He's just another entitled, southern, white guy with money. Maybe he was bullied a little for being a "fat goth kid." (His words, not mine.) But that doesn't mean he's justified in being a bully and a rapist.*

When explaining the *intersections of minority and privileged identities of the aggressor*, participants shared their attempt to understand the systemic oppressions their aggressor experiences in their sociocultural and contextual factors. For some participants, looking at these intersections facilitated the process of forgiveness while others attempted to have some level of empathy for aggressors sharing similar intersecting identities in the world.

Overall, the *aggressor's power and privilege* emerged as an important theme following the second-round analyses in explaining the experience and process of sexual violence. Participants shared the impact of the aggressor's *physical strength* in creating a safety risk and contributing to their inability to defend themselves at the time of the sexual violence. Most participants also shared the privileged identities and higher power of the aggressor's race as white and their gender as being male. They described the white man identity of their aggressor as "obvious" in holding more power than them. In addition, the *positional and social power* of the aggressor was explained by the aggressor's higher professional and expertise hierarchy, financial status, social acceptance, and access to means within the social and professional network the participants were a part of. Participants also considered the role of the *intersections of minority and privileged identities of the aggressor* as they created meaning from their experience. In other words, processing the sexual violence sometimes involved empathizing, explaining the aggressor's positionality, and attempting to forgive their aggressor.

Survivor's power and privilege. This second *subcategory* under **power and privilege** was created following the second-round analyses and refers to the participants' power and privilege in relation to their identities and the resulting encounters they had with the system. The *survivor's power and privilege subcategory* consisted of participants' voices relative to their experience with systemic oppression due to their minority identities, as well as the emotional burden associated with these encounters within the sociocultural and historical systems. This *subcategory* has a dimension of encounters with the system and a *property* of *emotional burden*.

Encounters with the system. This dimension was further clarified and defined as participants' encounters with "isms" and systemic oppression due to their minority identities. Participants discussed the racism, misogyny, sexism, homophobia, and other systemic and normative encounters they faced prior, during and after the sexual violence. All of these systemic encounters have impacted how participants viewed themselves and created meaning from their experience when navigating the journey after sexual trauma. Participants discussed their encounters with the system both individually as well as collectively with those whom they shared identities.

The following quotes from the second-round analyses confirmed the participants' encounter of "isms" that were specifically targeted at them. Nathan shared the impact of racist comments by his aggressor as he engaged in a healing process and created meaning from his encounter with sexual violence:

> **Nathan:** [long silence] Well, I remember that her [the aggressor] comments about me being, you know, a short Asian guy really made me dislike my height, and really, just maybe dislike being Asian. I also remember, um, I remember thinking the fact that she'd even bring up race was such a weird thing. Because what does it have to do with anything? But now it was like this, suddenly it was like this demerit on my life like it was a flaw. And when you see your race as something that's flawed. And, you know, a white person tells you that, you feel like you're abnormal or like the other. And, it's very difficult to pull yourself out of that space when you live in a state that's mostly white people. So, my healing process was affected because I was consistently surrounded by white people. And now I was consistently aware that I was, um, Asian, and I wasn't like them. And physically people see that and no matter how superficial or integrated into white culture I might be, it doesn't take away that my skin or my eye shape is different, if that makes sense. And it often left, so like tying that all back together, I would say that the fact or her power as a white woman and her ability to impose these negative feelings of my own race on to me negatively impacted my healing in a way where it's stagnated how I viewed myself in any positive light. Does that make sense?

Nathan goes on to explain the nuances of having a mixed-race background, his experiences with microaggressions, and at the same time the trust and strong connections that were established with close friends despite their race-based comments:

> **Nathan:** that [efforts to belong to white culture] becomes even more strange to navigate through when it comes to interpersonal relationships with other people, in just in general, like with friendships or romances because, you know, I feel like every friend I've ever had has always [made] some sort of like off-hand Asian comment, but at the same time I also know that every friend I've ever made stand up for me if they ever saw someone being racist towards me, and I do know that I have been fetishized by white people before, and simultaneously I also know that, like, I've also felt very ugly. So, like, it's, it's a weird. It's a really weird space to exist in.

Similarly, in connection with the artifact (poem) representing their journey after sexual trauma, Nichole also shared their fear that their skin color is associated with safety risks as well as the double burden of being a racial minority intersecting with their immigration status here in the United States:

> **Nichole:** um... a poem a while ago around the same time as the incident.... it was about, not about sexual trauma specifically, it was more about like this sort of fear that things happen to me because I'm in a brown body. Or that, like my having a brown body means that I can't have the same joys and connections as other people. But that's just not the case, so that the poem is really about like, um, (pause) I don't have to do anything to be a daughter. I am one. I don't have to do anything to be a granddaughter to my grandmother. I am one. Um (pauses) yeah. And the more I think about it, the more it's exactly like saying that my body is not an apology. Or it-It's sort of the argument for something of... so that's what I'm thinking of.

River, on the other hand, shared the sexist comments the aggressor made following the sexual violence that contributed the negative outcomes by forcing her to internalize the blame:

> **River:** yeah, it [sexual violence] didn't change anything [laughter] after the event happened, he [the aggressor] was exactly the same, so only then he got to call me a slut so it, I mean, it definitely made things worse in that way. And then I blamed myself. And 'what did I do?' Well, I was like 'I thought, doing this thing would, like, fix it.'

The gendered and sexualized socializations and expectations associated with the norms of the society were also connected with participants' sexual violence experiences. Nichole, as a gender non-binary identifying person, shared the intersections of others' views on their body and the encounter with sexual violence:

> **Nichole**: Yeah, I was like 'no, I don't. I don't need to be protected because I'm like a girl.' First of all, I'm not a girl. And don't relate to people who experience violence because they're women or something like that. I didn't- I maybe experienced it because I'm perceived as one or because I have the right genitals. But it did feel more like, um yeah, and maybe like the violence having happened because I was, um, perceived as having a certain sexuality and gender identification felt like an additional burn.

One participant shared the culture within the entertainment industry that contributed to the consistent encounter of unwanted sexual advances with co-workers. Tim Samson, who has experienced sexual violence from both men and women, in his poem, reflected on the culture in the entertainment industry that led to his multiple sexual violence encounters by highlighting what it means to be a minority "straight guy":

> *If I was gay, I woulda had my pick.*
> *Turns out I was just "the gayest straight guy I know" to everyone, just waiting for their sexual suspicions to be confirmed.*
> *Turns out queer doesn't mean I want to fuck you. #sorrynotsorry*

Moreover, during the second-round interviews there were multiple references to participants' experience with "isms" and the system collectively as members of an underrepresented group. These references confirmed and elaborated participants' disclosures during the first-round analyses. Some of these *collective experiences of "isms" and the system* were not specifically targeted towards the participants, however, they created a meaning about their identities by observing how others were treated. For instance, Tim Samson stated how he learned about code switching and oppressing his feminine side to fit into the social expectations of masculinity:

> **Tim Samson**: I grew up in a rural town in Northern [West] and it was, you know, I think we had one person of color in my entire high school, like it was very much like it was a homogeneous culture, like everybody, went to the same church [laughter] It was like we all like. It was very clearly defined, and there were a couple of kids who were like pretty obviously queer in some way. And they were bullied, you know. So, it was like you, either …'don't do that like' [laughter]. You just all in line and be like everybody else, and I was decent enough at that because I was good at sports.

In addition, Nathan explained that race-based assumptions and stereotypes of the attractiveness and masculinity of those identifying as Asian had impacted his self-image:

> **Nathan**: [silence] So the answer is, [long silence and hesitance] I am, as an Asian American man, I have often felt that I am not considered to be physically attractive, and I've often felt that my, I talked about this last time that my height plays a role in a lot of different things, and I've often felt that [silence] Asian men aren't necessarily seen as very masculine at least not in not in like a white Western kind of view.

> **Nathan:** And you know a white person tells you that ["a short Asian guy"] you feel like you're abnormal or like the other, and it's very difficult to pull yourself out of that space when you live in a state that's mostly white people. So, my healing process was affected because I was consistently surrounded by white people. And now I was consistently aware that I was, um, Asian, and I wasn't like them. And physically. People see that and no matter how superficial or integrated into white culture I might be, it doesn't take away that my skin or my eye shape is different, if that makes sense.

These collective and systemic encounters of "isms" impact the decisions of survivors to seek justice following the experience of sexual violence, and is intertwined with the aggressor's

privileged race and gender:

> **Nathan:** Yeah, because male sexual is already not taken nearly as seriously as female sexual assault. And at the same time, I think that [silence] I think that ethnic people are often considered scary to most white people. I mean, we can talk about like yellow peril or like how White women being raped was often the thing of like the cause for a lot of lynching, you know, like these types of things happen. So I think that just being a white woman who can kind of, she has a certain value, social value, and it's different than ethnic women. And please forgive me if that's ignorant because I could be completely wrong.

> **Nathan:** I feel like if I were, one scenario that I've often played in my head is, if this [sexual violence] were to happen again, and I did tell someone. I often wonder if my aggressor could flip it around and say, "that's not how it happened." And then it would just be a game of well, who's telling the truth? And I know that women go through this all the time, because I've seen court cases where men flip it around, and they're like, "no, it was woman's entire fault." And I think that's incredibly awful that we can just do that to someone and invalidate their feelings and these experiences that were forced upon them um…but then, as a man who has faced something like this, I also know that, like a woman [would] be believed over me specially a white woman.

In addition, Tim Samson explained how encounters with the system show up for individuals in a privileged space.

> **Tim Samson:** I mean I have a suspicion that, like most people are aware that they're stuck in a patriarchal system in this country and that I mean, I say most people, I think a lot of a lot of people that like obviously suffer the ill effects of the patriarchy like that are in poverty, or like what experiencing like racism or sexism or like. But yeah, the Patriarchy fucking sucks. But I think a lot of like people that live in a pretty privileged place are like, "oh, where that maybe something's not quite right" like "we're living in like this feels pretty good, but I'm pretty unfulfilled."

He further clarified the intersection of holding privileged identities and yet experiencing oppression.

> **Tim Samson:** ...and it [oppression]'s such a weird thing that, like oppression, or the folks in the from the privilege perspective like me, like, is absence of emotional freedom, I think, like the oppression is of emotions and of how we must perform and that is an oppression. And I think you know, it's sometimes difficult to communicate that, because it's not the same as like a trans kid in [rural state] is literally in danger of their life like and I'm not trying to equate the two, but, like it is...it is a legitimate of oppression.

In sum, the *survivor's encounters with the system*, experienced both individually and collectively with those identifying as minority group members, have negatively impacted participants' journeys following sexual trauma.

Emotional burden. The *property* of *emotional burden* under the *survivor's power and privilege* was felt by participants as they encounter the systems in their immediate and larger context. The *emotional burden* was supported by a dimension of conforming to advocacy. This dimension was created by merging two dimensions created during the first-round analysis: conforming to questioning and awareness to advocacy.

Conforming to advocacy. This dimension refers to participants' transition from conforming to the existing societal norms and systems to advocating for theirs and others' rights. The dimension of conforming to advocacy was defined by participants' experience of first questioning the existing systems and then gathering knowledge to then be able to advocate. During the second-round analysis, the dimension of conforming to advocacy was specifically confirmed by River's experiences of questioning feminine-based norms and socializations:

> **River:** ...'oh, so that's just a weird Southern thing' like 'that's part of the weird Southern culture of' like "Oh, don't make people uncomfortable." And I'm like, 'why? So?' It's like, maybe like question things and maybe like not afraid to like...because, like most of the time the people that you're not supposed to make uncomfortable [are]

usually the abusers. So, it's like, 'why, why shouldn't we be making them uncomfortable?' They sure made me uncomfortable so...

Tim Samson discussed his intentional shift to <u>advocacy</u> instead of conforming to stereotypical masculine behaviors when he is around other men who display these behaviors:

> **Tim Samson:** and it I just I see that more now that I know what I'm looking for, see it more and more, and then where they just they run and hide from their feelings in ways that are just like so pervasive. And I can do it myself, like when I get around men, I do the same behavior like, I'm working against that, but like I tend to like, get more physical space, I tend to like talk about sports, or, you know, talk about that. But if I can model, maybe a different version of that [masculinity], like. Maybe I can help open door for somebody else. That's something I'm reconciling with right now is my own bravery when it comes to that yeah...

Moreover, Nathan shared his goal of participating in this study as a way to advocate and be a "voice" for men sexual trauma survivors:

> **Nathan:** And another meaning I've made of it [the journey after sexual violence] is [silence] understanding [that] this happens to all people, and all people deserve our empathy and sympathy when these types of problems arise, and we as a society, and, as you know, like in in America, as a culture, we have to really take these things seriously, and also stigmatize it on all fronts like even for women, for men, for people of color, for people who are white for all people. I don't dislike any people, and... this [sexual violence] happens to all cultures, all people, all races. And this isn't just like something that happens to one group of people. And I'm just really glad that I was able to be a part of this [study] in a way where I give voice to my people, to people like me.

However, Nathan also explained the survivor's *emotional burden* when he expresses his feelings of failing to make a difference by advocating for himself as well as others:

> **Nathan:** [silence]I don't want to seem negative um [silence] but when I first contacted you and wanted to be a part of this [study]. I said how I wanted to give a voice to men who had gone through sexual trauma, and who had [silence] who may have been embarrassed or may have been misrepresented or I wanted to show that it happens, and that it was okay to talk about. But ever since I went back into a dark place, and I started thinking...I've started to think that no one really cares [voice starts shaking] about men's sexual trauma, and that even if I do speak up or talk about it, that socially and culturally in we, at least in the Western, like American world, I don't think we really care about those people. I don't think we care about men like that. And it's been very difficult to accept, um, but it's kind of what I've come to the conclusion of.

> **Nathan:** and I feel like there are so many... There are so many different things that that we're trying to make better in the world. They're like all these different metaphorical wars that we're fighting like for social justice. And there's so many that are going on that not everyone can invest all their time into all of them. So I think that when we think about sexual trauma or sexual assault towards men, or just sexual assault towards anyone in general, we usually give it more towards women or feminine identities. And I think that [silence] that's fair I think that women have it rougher than men do and even though it really hurts my feelings that no one most people probably don't care about me as much. I, I understand it. And it's something that I feel like I just need to get over.

This discouragement and the *emotional burden* of engaging in advocacy was evident in Nathan's poem addressing the exhaustion and feeling of helplessness because he felt invisible as others addressed sexual trauma in educational settings:

> *...Professor asks why, wonders why I'm suddenly distant. I tell them how some might be afraid of me. He tells me to get thicker skin. Now I feel like I'm overreacting. Maybe I was*
> *overreacting with Hailey, too. Maybe it's all an overreaction, I just need thicker skin.*
> *I keep coming to class. Quieter each day. Less enthusiastic. I lay my head on the desk, withdraw*
> *myself from conversations. One lecture, my professor speaks on the concept of toxic masculinity. Someone raises their hand, claims that toxic masculinity is innate to men, that men*
> *suppress their emotions due to social constructs. I hear Hailey again. How she said it can't happen to men. My professor and I lock eyes, prompting them to call my name, asking if*
> *I have something to add. I open my mouth and say:*
> *'Yeah, that sounds about right.'*

However, despite periodic discouragement regarding advocacy, Nathan shared his determination to "make a difference" by giving voice to male survivors of sexual violence:

> **Nathan:** It [participating in this study] feels so small that I'm not entirely sure it makes a difference. And I really want it to make a difference, but I just don't know if it does. And the reason why I'm here is because I still want it to make a difference. And I saw faith in it.

On advocacy regarding race and *racial identity*, Nathan shared that he often uses classroom lessons to educate others about diversity and culture so those from privileged racial identities can learn about the cultures of those in underrepresented groups:

> **Nathan:** Especially as more interracial relationships are becoming more and more prominent, I have sort of a view, my Asian ethnicity, my Asian American nature as a positive thing, as something that I think that I should own, and I should be very confident especially as of as of lately, ever since finishing up the semester, I've been very confident about talking about Asian American struggles, about doing Asian American literature for classrooms like I feel like it's really important to talk about that stuff [high pitch; matter of fact expression with high energy].

At the same time, Nathan questioned the effectiveness of his advocacy about racial identity and creating awareness of the rich culture of underrepresented groups:

> **Nathan:** what's been helpful is that I feel like I give people perspective and them obtaining that perspective typically gives them a little bit of insight. I'm not always sure if it resonates because I think that ethnicity and race is a lived experience, and no matter how much someone informs another person, it doesn't, you're never going to know fully.

In summary, participants highlighted the survivor's *emotional burden* associated with questioning and advocating to change the culture surrounding sexual violence. Specifically, discouragements related to advocacy have negatively impacted participants' wellbeing. Participants shared their continued interest in speaking out against the social norms that silenced their voice, and in bringing inclusivity into discussions regarding their minority identities and sexual violence.

In general, the **survivor's power and privilege** emerged based on the experience of the participants who found themselves in a lesser position of power due to their minority identities. Lesser power and privilege was connected to participants' experience with sexual violence in that these power differences with the aggressor contributed to the sexual violence and/or the "isms" participants experienced following the sexual violence. This category was supported by the <u>encounters with the system dimension</u> and *emotional burden property*.

Overall, the **category of power and privilege**, focused on participants' perceptions and conceptualizations of the socially- and contextually informed power and privilege they themselves and their aggressor held. Participants discussed the *aggressor's power and privilege* in relation to the aggressor's *positional and social power, privileged race and gender identities, physical strength,* and *intersection of minority and privileged identities of the aggress*or. In addition, participants discussed the power and privilege they held prior, during and after the sexual violence. Under the *survivor's power and privilege*, participants discussed their encounters with the system and the *emotional burden* as they transform themselves from conforming to advocacy. The less **power and privilege** participants held in their society due to their identities and social positions, the more they faced challenges and emotional burdens of navigating these systems. These encounters with "isms" have led participants to question the existing **sociocultural contexts and socialization**, work on developing their awareness about **power and privilege**, and advocate both for themselves and others, leading to survivor's *emotional burden*.

Trauma response

The definition and conceptualization of the **trauma response** category, previously named **responding to trauma**, remained the same after the second-round analyses. The *subcategories: somatic responses, emotional responses, psychological responses, and behavioral responses* also remained the same and their definitions unchanged. However, the names of *physical distance from the perpetrator*, previously a *property* under the *behavioral responses*, and *empathy,* previously a *property* under the *psychological responses*, were changed to *maintaining physical boundaries* and *empathy towards others,* respectively. Their definitions and conceptualizations, however, remained the same. In addition, the dimension of naming and normalizing, under *psychological responses,* was reconceptualized as a PROCESS RECOGNIZING SEXUAL ENCOUNTER AS VIOLENCE to connect the

PROCESS of SHIFT IN UNDERSTANDING OF CONSENT with **trauma response**. Moreover, a new PROCESS was created under **psychological responses**: INTERNALIZING BLAME TO EXTERNALIZING BLAME. Not all participants revisited their response to trauma and no specific guiding question was asked on this topic during the second-round interview. Below are the quotes regarding **trauma response** as discussed by participants during the second-round analyses.

Somatic responses. One participant in particular shared the nature of the somatic trauma responses ranging from immediate to ongoing, stating that, despite all the intentional effort and personal growth, she still anticipates experiencing panic attacks during initial sexual interactions with new partners:

> **Sophie:** it would be very fair for me to expect myself to have more reactions again, more like trauma reactions, should I be intimate with somebody in the future. And, so that song had this pattern of like this idea of like I'm gaining insight, and I'm making headway, and no matter how much headway I see myself making, I still end up finding myself getting tripped up back in the same visceral space or head space, and then it's. you know, I think it's kind of like a baseline anxiety and security on my own. And then it's definitely, (pause) then triggered in like initial, like sexual interactions,

Nathan, in his poem, also reiterated the *somatic responses* immediately prior and right after his encounter with sexual violence by describing his trauma response experience as "freeze":

> *Hailey told me about what he did to her, how she never wanted it and no one believed her.*
> *She said how I was lucky because that sort of thing can't happen to boys.*
> *She described her turmoil, each word making my hands ball into trembling fists.*
> *Then she touched my thigh, rubbed the inner seam of my jeans with her polished fingernails before pouncing on me in the passenger seat. Her teeth bit my lip, tongue stuffed*
> *down my throat to where I couldn't speak. It's fight, flight, or freeze. I froze. Her weight slammed my head against the window so hard I imagined it cracking like ice.*
> *She pulled away, rubbing my cheek with her thumb. She said I was really handsome, that I had a cute dimple on the side of my face when I grinned, a sturdy build she felt could*

> handle her. I was silent, wide-eyed, short, heavy breaths escaping from my lips, my chest heaving with unease. Her eyes narrowed as she began to pat the center of my pants, pecking my neck. I
> said nothing. She noticed that I was shaking, shivering as if I had been outside in the cold for the past hour. She poked me, her big, blue eyes slanted in a glare. She asked if I liked her. I responded with
> stillness. She stopped straddling me, lifted herself, scoffed like I was a disgusting creature.

For participants, like Nathan, who experienced "freeze" response to trauma during the sexual violence encounter, *somatic responses* were experienced as moments of silence and not being able to assert themselves. For others, like Sophie, the *somatic responses* were described as active trauma responses that occur on an ongoing basis as they experience triggering events.

Emotional responses. Some participants shared the anger and *shame and guilt* they feel as they continue their journey following the sexual violence. Anger was expressed as a righteous anger that was felt by participants after recalling the lack of control over their own body while the sexual violence was happening. *Shame and guilt*, on the other hand, had multiple sources. Participants shared experiencing guilt for their perceived role leading to and during the sexual violence. Shame was also associated with anticipating triggering sexual encounters that potentially could lead to panic attacks.

Anger. This dimension under *emotional responses* was discussed by participants as a cycle that kept happening as they created meaning from their sexual trauma experience. During the second-round analyses, Tim Samson shared the dimension of anger by noticing the shift from feeling angry to recognizing the righteousness of the anger he felt when remembering how the sexual violence experiences transpired:

> **Tim Samson:** I got angry. I was writing it and it's something that we talked before I'm like I don't feel anger. I don't feel mad. But then, sort of like letting my memory sort of walk back there, I found myself being like that time I was just so out of control of my own anything like that I was just desperate to work, you know, so like I would do anything for work, and you know I wasn't in control of my own body, and people were

> telling me like "this is how, your voice has to sound like" and it's all sort of wrapped in this odd framework of "you're lucky to be here" and so like "you just sort of jump through the hoops, and you don't really question it." aha...surprisingly, I was really surprised how angry I got as I was writing it [the poem to represent his journey following sexual trauma]. It's good to feel anger, I think, and that's difficult for me to say out loud. So in that way it's very meaningful as a means of expression.... I can access that anger. And I know that it's not going to destroy me in a way that like is really I don't know [silence].
>
> **Tim Samson:** um...I'm angry that people treated my body as though it wasn't mine. but more than anything, just that time, for, like nothing was mine, like I. Everything was just like on a conveyor belt that somebody else is pushing the button and a real I didn't realize, even though I followed my dreams, and, like I, I ostensibly chose to do this career in retrospect. It doesn't feel like a choice at all. It's not like I became the mascot for the[my] department, because I was good at [previous profession], and my professor wanted to sort of hold me up and say, "Look, look at this one" and then same thing like once I got to [metropolitan city] it was like some people wanted to hold me up for their own benefit, and a lot of people just want to have sex with me...um... and there's even shame saying that because that's in a weird as a privilege statement in a weird sort of way, because but it's not a privilege, in the sense of how it actually feels as a privilege in the sense of the patriarchy.

This anger Tim Samson felt towards having less control over choices he could make about his own body while the sexual violence was happening shifted to righteous anger as he reflected more about his experience:

> **Tim Samson:** And it was just like picturing myself like in the way that it felt. It all happened in front of people like that feeling of just being trapped like. "Oh, of course you can do that. Of course, you can do that like we're on the lights around us. We're on stage. We're like, of course, of course, I'm lucky to be here" like in that. You know how easy it is when certain structures are in place to for people to just [get] really harmed. And they can't fight back.

This righteous anger was reflected in Tim Samson's artwork, a poem representing his journey of healing from sexual trauma. The poem partly reads as:

> *Of course, you can grope me. Grab my ass. Of course. Tell me you want to lick the veins in my abs. Of course. It's all in good fun. It's just the culture. After all, aren't I lucky to be here? Of course, you can tell me you just know I'm gay – and you'd be happy to help me get there. So gentle, so well-intentioned. Of course, you can grab my dick in front of people. What am I going to do? I'm lucky to be here.*

Shame and guilt. Participants discussed *shame and guilt,* a *property* under the *emotional responses,* as an experience that happens intermittently when they feel triggered and display active *somatic responses.* Sophie specifically described her "frustration" about anticipating "panic attacks" when planning to establish new romantic relationships involving sexual activity:

> **Sophie:** it would be very fair for me to expect myself to have more reactions again, more like trauma reactions, should I be intimate with somebody in the future ... I guess in this moment it feels, it kind of represents frustration that I feel, like, I have that even with growth (pause) and personal development that (pause) history is still very much alive in me. It just keeps coming up. yeah, it's still present. yeah, I mean, reliably frustrating and embarrassing when it happens.

Nathan, Tim Samson and River added the *shame and guilt* they feel because of their perceived responsibility leading to and/or following the sexual violence. This guilt is connected to the socializations on sexuality and masculinity that led to thinking that they had contributed to the sexual violence or had been complicit when the sexual violence was happening, as well as the guilt they felt for not speaking up against the *positional and social power* of their aggressors:

> **River:** I felt like it [sexual violence] was like, my only chance to get back in [to her peer group] and it just made me feel really pathetic for lack of a better word. Because it was a part of me that's like 'am I just like sweating myself out so I can like hang out with my friends, because that's gross with me to do.' Why am I doing that?

> **Nathan:** I've been being open with my feelings. I've been trying to not feel so guilty all the time. I know one thing that my therapist said is that I seem to have like a massive guilt complex... it's [the sexual violence] one of the bigger reasons I feel really guilty, but I wouldn't say it's the only reason, I think, that there has been a lot in my life that I've experienced that may make me feel guilty, and this was just a really bad experiences that added on to all that... my mom was very religious...she would often, she saw most sexual acts [as] something that need to be very private and are. It's like shameful. And I remember one thing that she used to kind of really [silence] try to teach, I guess, like impose was that if there wasn't any feelings or some sort of any feelings, or intimate romance, there shouldn't be anything sexual going on.

> **Tim Samson**: And a lot of people just want to have sex with me, um, and there's even shame saying that because that's in a weird as a privilege statement in a weird sort of way, because but it's not a privilege, in the sense of how it actually feels as a privilege in the sense of the patriarchy...there is something lovely about getting it like I get why this [inability to name and recognize sexual violence as it happens] happens, and I know what, how I, my role in that, and I feel some shame around that. And I can sort of think about why do I feel shame? And I cannot feel shame that I feel shame, you know.

In his poem, Nathan also added his experience of sadness witnessing social justice movements such as the #MeToo Movement that mostly focused on women survivors of sexual trauma:

> *I started the semester off with it* [sexual violence] *in the back of my mind. I tried not to, but somedays it was all I thought about. There was an assault march I got stuck in while heading to my poetry*
> *class. The participants held signs, waved flags, chanted how they believed survivors. Me too. But then I remembered that it can't happen to boys so I ran to the bathroom, cried, wore sunglasses so*
> *no one would see, thanked god the mask mandate covered the emotions on my face.*

The most common experiences of *emotional responses* were anger and *shame and guilt*. Anger often shifted to righteous anger that helped participants to externalize the blame and help them set their boundaries. The *shame and guilt* have been associated with participants' perceived accountability during the sexual violence or related to continued experiences of *somatic responses* to sexual trauma.

Psychological responses. This *subcategory* was related to the participants' understanding and meaning of the sexual trauma encounter and events that transpired along with that experience. Among the existing dimensions under the *subcategory* of *psychological response*, during second-round interviews self-worth was revisited by participants as an important component in their **trauma response**. Two participants shared the views and behavioral measures that helped them maintain a positive outlook on themselves:

> **Nathan:** yes, to elaborate on that, one of the feelings that I've often felt is if I don't have a goal that I'm pursuing, or if I don't have some something that I'm doing that that that makes me feel like I'm being productive. I start to think negatively about myself. And then I think back to the moments, and then it starts to, it just starts to shift my mode and just my perspective on life.
>
> **Nathan:** Ever since I started seeing therapy, I started like writing positive affirmations. I've been being open with my feelings.
>
> **Tim Samson:** I'm really proud of myself, I mean, that's a, I guess that's meaning like, it really, it would have been so easy to not work on healing. Let's just follow the career, continue doing what I'm doing like have that sort of vague dissatisfaction. But I'm not. I had to want to do the work and I think I could have phoned it into for counseling, so I could have done like the surface level. But like but I didn't. I work really hard really unpack my shit. I see counselors. I've seen several counselors. I get mental health counseling regularly, like I've done that work…
>
> **Nichole:** (long pause) I think mostly, um, I got to show myself that I'm…(pause), on the one end, that I'm a really resilient person, and, uh, I don't have to be afraid of bad things happening like not only do I have like a lot of the internal resources that are necessary for taking on a healing journey, but also that (pause) the people that I need find me. Not even that I find them where that like, I choose them, because sometimes they choose me, but I always felt like the universe has cared for me in that way.

Nathan also revisited the importance of actively working on changing negative thoughts and self-talk to the positive to maintain a positive self-worth:

> **Nathan:** I think, that filling your time with activities or hobbies, or personal goals helps you overcome thinking about negative things. especially when you have like spiraling thoughts that kind of lead back to one thing and like, whenever I'm about to go into those, those downward spirals of thoughts. I always feel it's best to just not think about it and do something else like a different activity. So, I've taken up a lot of hobbies too.

One participant also reiterated the importance of *authenticity* as he navigates the journey following sexual violence. Tim Samson stated that part of the healing and meaning-making process was allowing himself to be congruent with all parts of his identities:

> **Tim Samson:** yeah, And I think you know, that's when I think about identity, like I have so many of them. And it's so fun. And it's so special. And we all do [have a lot of identities]. And as I'm growing and interacting with the world differently, I'm finding that my identities are feeling more and more authentic. And that feeling like "something's not quite right", is revealing what's not quite right about that is that I was

performing like 'I'm performing what I'm supposed to do.' This is how I how I fit in society, and wonderfully and maybe surprisingly as I'm getting more comfortable with these very personal identities and letting them be like ones that I perform, I actually feel more collectivist because I'm not trying to uphold some sort of individualist mantle. I'm just here. I am interacting for the better it meant for the. My intention is to make the world better, which means interacting, which means interacting authentically and so yeah, all of these sorts of difficult things, they're and they're all difficult every time you sort of reconcile with something.

In summary, under *psychological responses*, participants talked about the importance of shifting from internalizing blame to externalizing blame as a step towards the healing journey from sexual trauma. Moreover, participants talked about the shift towards positive self-worth and *authenticity* as they navigate life with trauma.

Behavioral responses. This *subcategory* was primarily revisited regarding participants' perspectives on the value of positive *body awareness and image, therapy* and *journaling and creative outlets*. While the conceptualization and naming remained the same for *therapy*, journaling and writing was changed to *journaling and creative outlets* with the same conceptualization to give room for creative efforts outside of journaling and writing.

Therapy. Two participants specifically discussed the importance or potential importance of *therapy*. Nathan, who started seeing a therapist after the first-round interview, disclosed that attending therapy had helped him to address the negative self-talk and guilt he had been experiencing. Sophie, on the other hand, shared her hope that focusing on sexual trauma in therapy would yield a good outcome in her healing journey:

> **Nathan:** Ever since [the first-round interview] I started seeing therapy, I started like writing positive affirmations. I've been being open with my feelings. I've been trying to not feel so guilty all the time.

> **Sophie:** I guess in this moment it feels it kind of represents frustration that I feel. Like, I have that even with growth (pause) and personal development that (pause) history is still very much alive in me. And I haven't done therapy work specifically on that, and I would expect that to make a difference.

Body awareness and image. Participants also revisited the importance of body awareness and image as they explore their identities and create a meaning to their sexual trauma. Specifically, Nichole discussed the importance of having a positive body image as part of owning one's identity and making positive progress towards healing from sexual trauma:

> **Nichole:** But I'm just out here having a body, and some people think that that means they can use it…I don't have to prove it. And um (pause) my, my body was intended for like really beautiful things. Period.

> **Nichole:** the first one is, it was a sort of flow song that I found on the Instagram a while ago, and she, this person just creates, uh she just sings whatever, like improvises on themes, and posts them on Instagram. But the refrain of the songs, 'my body is not an apology'. And it's just the catchiest little thing, too. So, I like sing it to myself sometimes. So, like really grounding rhythm. My body is not an apology. My body, uh, born to be free! I think there's some, I'm missing some words that I'm not quoting it exactly, but that's just so true. It's just like the thing that the thing that enables me to move through the world. Yeah. And I don't know, I also think of this song like when I have some friends- I have a lot of friends with body image stuff and with sexual trauma, and listening to the way that they talk about their bodies as if what it looks like or what has happened to in the past has, is some sort of value statement of what it's capable of is heartbreaking to me, and I just like to remind them that, like I don't look at them and think like something's wrong with their body. I think, like 'I'm so glad that you are in a body so that I can meet up with you, like I know where to find you because you have a body.' It's kind of like all that I see it being for just the… it's a relational tool. And it's, yeah. It's like so sad that relationship gets broken by certain experiences. But that's what that song reminds me of.

In reference to celebrating and having a positive body image, Nichole shared @thebengsons's Instagram handle and link for the "my body is not an apology" song as one of the artworks representing their journey after sexual violence. The lyrics of the song, from the Instagram website, are as follows:

> *My body is not an apology*
> *My body was born beloved and free*
> *My body was made for nobody but me*
> *My body is not an apology*
> **hmmhmmhmm**
> *My body is not an apology*

> *My body was born beloved and free*
> *My body is for nobody but me*
> *My body is not an apology*
> **hmmhmmhmm**

Similarly, Tim Samson shared the body awareness he continues to develop as he learns more about the power and privileges associated with certain body types:

> **Tim Samson:** I haven't really thought about my body size, like I thought about my body as like a a vessel of sexual trauma. But like I've not thought about like." Oh, I'm little like I can think I'm a little guy. I'm a for guy" like, and it's sort of a joke but it's also a privilege like I mean, not in every space, but in a lot of spaces.

He also stated that continuing to explore his body image outside of the traumatic sexual experience has been helpful.

Journaling and creative outlets. In discussing the role of art in their journey following sexual violence, participants talked about the importance of writing and engaging in creative outlets in processing the traumatic experience. These creative outlets were not only used to express their emotional reactions and perspectives but also to express their pains and views of their encounter with the world:

> *River:* River: ... I think it's [writing about the sexual trauma] good because it's...one, I want it to be something that I can one day share with other people, so other people can read it and it's also good for me, and like I thought it would be more upsetting because I mean, I write about all sorts of things that have happened to me...um...like friends dying, and all sorts of things. And I thought this would be more upsetting for me to write but it actually wasn't.
>
> **Nathan:** ... I play four instruments. I play guitar. I play ukulele. I consider singing [with] an instrument and I also play a little bit of banjo...I wrote a song that's kind of...it's about me and my brother, and how we open up about our experiences that we're kind of shared and overlapped. And I feel like that might be thematically fitting to maybe submit as the art. so those are the two things my poetry and kind of like my letters, which I feel like are very similar. The poem is a little is a little different. The poem is more of a recollection of the events that transpired and just different feelings, different negative feelings. I was thinking it's a far more negative piece of art. I think. It kind of tells a small little narrative. It's a long for a poem, though, which is why, I feel a little insecure about like sharing it right away, which I feel like I need to edit just as a writer.

Tim Samson: Whenever I write, and I do. I used to do a lot of writing. I still write from time to time like I can tell when I'm writing poetry that gets me going because I'll just like, and you'll see there's a place where there's just like a chunk [chuckles]. It's like furiously typing like. And I'll start like repeating phrases, and I'll start like echoing myself, and sort of like rhyming within myself and because it just like this sort of like the physical manifestation sort of, but that I feel somatically sort of bubbles out through my fingertips.

Nichole: I wrote a poem a while ago. Around the same time as the incident. But it was about, not about sexual trauma specifically. It was more about like this sort of fear that things happen to me because I'm in a brown body. Or that, like my having a brown body means that I can't have the same joys and connections as other people. But that's just not the case, so that the poem is really about like, um, (pause) I don't have to do anything to be a daughter. I am one. I don't have to do anything to be a granddaughter to my grandmother. I am one. Um (pauses) yeah. And the more I think about it, the more it's exactly like saying that my body is not an apology. Or it-It's sort of the argument for something [like that].

In sum, during the second-round interview, participants revisited aspects of **trauma responses** that were still significantly shaping their journey following the sexual violence experience. Not all *subcategories* under this **category** were represented in this second-round analyses. Participants mostly discussed the salient nature of somatic trauma response ranging from immediate to ongoing and *emotional responses* mainly with the shift towards righteous anger and the continuity of *feeling shame and guilt*. Participants also discussed the importance of working on maintaining positive self-worth by focusing on affirmations and positive self-talk. *Therapy* was also revisited as an important aspect of developing insights into the impact of the sexual violence and taking actions to minimize these impacts.

Disclosure

This **category** and the *subcategories* of **disclosure** (*intrapersonal considerations of disclosure* and *interpersonal outcomes of disclosure*) remained the same following the second-round analyses. The following quotes further elaborated the *property* of *purpose of disclosure* under the *intrapersonal considerations of disclosure:*

> **River:** …and I feel like that makes not like that. It makes the experience okay, or anything. But I feel like I'm using it for good.
>
> **Nathan:** I think that the meaning that I make is to one be one of the few people who took steps into making it more normalized and making it more open to talk about, to showing that there is like data that that represents these types of people to give, giving people like me a voice. That's been one of the meanings that I made of it.

Under the *interpersonal outcomes of disclosure, social support* was confirmed by Tim Samson's experience of receiving support from his partner upon disclosure of his gender identity:

> **Tim Samson:** And it's been really I feel very free within myself for the first time, like, well, very fortunate. I have a super supportive partner like, "hey, I think I might be queer." She's like "Okay," "Think you might be, too."

Moreover, Tim Samson and River shared the importance of having a sense of community and support within their friendship group as they engage in the process of healing from the sexual violence:

> **Tim Samson:** and having a community of people who like want me to do that, you know, do that work. It's really like one of the artifacts of the patriarchy for me is that I have a hard time looking for help like I'll go to therapy but like that's the therapy space, like in my social spaces, I have a hard time being like 'I'm having a hard time' and just having people around me who are like "looks like you need some help" 'I think I do' is really… it's nice to be held accountable in a loving [and] caring sort of way like that…. It's such an abundance. I could call ten people right now, and I know they would pick up, and I know they would care even though we might not be like best friends, get together every day, these are people that I have emotional connections with I trust them. They trust me. We don't care that we're not perfect.
>
> **River:** …one of my good friends recently, he said something, and I was like 'you know, so hang out with him [the aggressor] anymore? And my friend was like "No, I might see him once a year or something", and then like I told him, and my friend was just like "oh, well, I won't be seeing him once a year anymore." 'No? Well, thank you. I appreciate that.' He's like "I have no clue" but I'm like 'well, it's a long time to like figure it out, but I was like that. That's the thing' and he's like "I'm really afraid. Sorry." I'm like 'it's okay…[laughter] you [are] the good one' And it's like 'I don't blame you for being friends with them, because, like, you don't know.'

Friends who were able to relate to the experience of the participants from a shared minority identity perspective have also been helpful to participants as they attempt to find comfort against systemic oppression:

> **Christina:** A lot of my friends are straight and white, which I am not straight or wide, but half white, and so when I guess when they were supporting me, they were doing it in the best way that they could, but support groups don't always know how to be the best if they can't relate. So even though they were very supportive, and they were very…they got me through everything. So that definitely was great. But I feel like one of the people who was able to support me more, she moved. how rude! But she is also she's half Filipino and so I was able to talk to her a little bit more, not only about like my trauma, but the other things that were happening in my life. And since I felt more supported in those other areas because she was able to relate. And when she talked to me about what had happened to me, I knew it wasn't coming from a very outsidery perspective if that makes sense. So even though she wasn't physically around, and I didn't get to talk to her as much, she was still, like, very foundational in the support. Just because of her, I guess, knowledge, we see this systemic basically black and white way of thinking. But even without realizing it, like our friends and family will have that way of thinking, too.

Similarly, Sophie shared that friends have been helpful in navigating secondary trauma:

> **Sophie:** um, talking with friends…mhmm…and it's this kind of fine line of talking with friends without, while, you know, respecting HIPAA and all of those pieces too.

On the other hand, participants reported *victim questioning* as a detrimental experience during their journey following sexual violence:

> **Nichole:** Yeah, I remember like getting questions like, 'Okay, but what did you... how were you...' I was like, no, I don't want to answer these questions. (laughs) It's awful.

Similarly, in her essay on the journey following sexual violence, River noted how her friends had questioned her experience of that trauma:

> *Once I could name it, I could box it up and put it on a shelf. It could live outside my body and I could finally tell it to people in a way it made sense. Some friends were skeptical: "But like, he didn't have a gun to your head."*
> *I had to tell them; "just because he wasn't about to murder me doesn't mean it's not rape." Because I know there's a gray area that this situation falls into. If I was to stand up in front of a jury, he would never be convicted and I would be slut shamed. This is one reason why victims don't speak up, they don't think anything will*

come of it, especially not anything good. It doesn't matter how many people I chose to sleep with; before and after...those were choices. Steven wasn't a choice.

Participants discussed the importance of connecting with others to get *social support*. However, the continuity of these *social support* systems can be a concern in some cases. For example, Nathan discussed how losing relationships also negatively impacted their **trauma response**. In his poem he shared how losing a new friend became a trigger:

> *I tried to move on, made lots of jokes, attempted to make friends, thought I had. One girl and I talked*
> *daily before class. Typical pleasantries, inoffensive small talk. Until she pulls me aside, tells me she wants to stop talking. She knows guys mistake kindness. Claims she has a boyfriend and hopes*
> *she's not sending the wrong signals. I swallow, gulp, wondering if she felt how Hailey felt. Now all I can think about is Hailey. begin to wonder if I scare women like Hailey scared me. I feel guilty, dumb, monstrous, like a dark shadow of the dread cast on others. I message my professors telling them I'd rather not participate anymore. I don't want anyone uncomfortable. I schedule an appointment with one professor, ask if I can stop coming to class so I don't make that girl afraid.*

Overall, the category of **disclosure** was revisited by participants in terms of their *purpose for disclosing* the sexual violence, and their altruistic motive to help others and give a voice to those who may not otherwise be able to speak out. In addition, participants discussed the importance of *social support* from their partners, friends, and professional groups as they navigate daily challenges and trauma responses.

Moments of relief

Following the second-round analyses, the **moments of relief and empowerment** was renamed as **moments of relief**, however, its definition remained the same. In addition, its dimension of specific moments of relief to recognition of overall personal growth was merged into the *subcategories* of *internal relief* and *external relief.* The experiences of **moments of** relief were described by participants as important factors to help them gain hope and provide evidence that healing could happen for them.

Two participants were able to clearly point out that the *internal relief* was associated with relief from sexual trauma while the *external relief* was related to relief from the systemic oppression they experienced due to their minority identities:

> **Christina:** the moments of relief that I felt from the system was more of, actually, I feel understood in that my basic human needs are going to be met, I guess, or at least like my medical needs will be met whereas, and that's like very external, whereas, like healing from this [sexual] trauma that was very internal, that was a lot of me not blaming myself not finding or not sitting in my anger. I guess so it even though, yes, I am angry at the system I would like it to change. It was very like external. I felt like, 'oh, if I don't like this, I can't, or if I don't like this doctor, I can go to another one. If I don't like this therapist, I can find another one.' If I don't like me, that sucks. And I'm stuck with me. So it's more of almost I have to find a way to heal with the trauma because I've been used to dancing around doctors and kind of just fitting the role that's needed as the patient. But I can't. I can't just not like myself.... So, finding then, that like internal validation, I think it's a lot harder... I mean, honestly, just as a human race like we are very critical of ourselves. So yeah, yeah, it's just very external versus internal healing.

> **Tim Samson:** Talking about the sexual trauma and healing from it. It's a really insular space within myself like it feels like it's mine that it's in here [pointing at his body] and the pain is like it is private pain, I mean...the reason that it [sexual violence] happened to me in the first place, is because of structures, but, like the subjective experience of it is mine. I can, because I'm talking about it sort of like feeling myself do this [closed arms] and so that feels, when I get relief from that, it's a very somatic experience where I can just be in my body and let it just and just exist...and I think that when I feel those moments of relief from the patriarchal systems, it's more of like a [holds arms up and wide] and less of a hmm [closed arms and body]. I could only sort of describe it in somatic terms. But there is a, the feeling that I get when I think about what I can sort of live through this [sexual trauma] all again like it, it's a yuck in the pit of my stomach, like I feel shame. And when I think about how far I've come and how much I recovered from that like, it's a loosening of shame. But it's not like a happy feeling. It's like a 'Yeah, that's not dogging me so much anymore. That's not like really making me like, it's not ruining my day.' There's not a lot of joy in it, I think, even in the relief, there's not like happiness. It's like the happiness has come from the exploration of identity that's come round in that healing. So they're related, but like the actual, if I look the assault in the eye, and I really like allow myself to think about where I'm at on that journey, it's absence of pain. [It] doesn't mean presence of happiness. It's just less bad, and it's allowed other happiness to come in which is nice.

One participant, however, described the **moments of relief** from both the sexual trauma and systemic oppression as internal experiences of freedom that helped develop positive self-worth and image:

> **Nathan:** So, I think that both are incredibly freeing... when you heal from sexual trauma, you become kind of a you. You start to piece yourself back together. If that makes sense, and when you're able to also own your identity, you're able to piece yourself back together in a different sense. does that make sense? Um, and I think that healing from sexual trauma helps me reclaim a [long silence] a lot of my worth, I suppose, and also...the moments of [relief] from the racial aspect also helps me feel complete, too.

Similarly, Nichole and Sophie shared the interrelatedness of the relief from the systemic oppression and moments of relief from sexual trauma:

> **Nichole:** um (pause) when I say that it [moments of relief from sexual trauma] feels like a category inside the other kind [moments of relief from systemic oppression]. It's like, um, when I'm feeling, you know, those moments of freedom from oppression so to speak reminds me that I have been, I have been freed from a type of it too.

> **Sophie:** (long pause) Um, (pause) I would say that I definitely have more of a (pause) I found myself to be a lot more, um, like triggered and like have, like panic attacks and hyperventilating when I'm initially intimate with men versus with women. And that is independent of any of their behavior. So definitely, I feel like it's hard to say if it's because I feel more accepted by another female or non-male person, or if it's because the trauma was with a male, so it's hard to pull those two pieces apart for sure. But that's where I would, you know, that's where I guess there's most notable, um, relief.

Collectively, there seems to be a shared experience of participants experiencing moments of relief from both sexual trauma and systemic oppression. Moments of relief from the sexual violence were more internal and emerged from experiences of internal peace, while relief from oppression was related to participants' engagement in inclusive social settings that allow them to exist equally with those in the dominant culture.

Internal relief. This *subcategory* of **moments of relief** was defined by the participants' experience of "internal peace" and hope as well as an experience of relief from "pain" that was caused by the sexual trauma they have endured. Some participants shared that these moments of *internal relief* were specific incidents and realizations that healing is possible, and that there was hope that they could heal from sexual trauma:

> **Christina:** So, the picture I had sent you was the one of my two best friends, and I watching the sunset over [West Coast] back home for me. And for me, that was really healing, because it was probably the first time in years, I truly felt at piece like there is no other worries in the world, that everything was fine. Everything was good just in that moment, like, it's basically perfect. And yeah, so that that was kind of the basis of like how I was feeling it. That was also the first time in many years I celebrated my birthday.

> **Nathan:** and [silence] I guess [silence] I'm not happy that I was assaulted, and I'm not happy that I had all these racial components to it but I am glad to know that, like at least some people find Asian guys attractive [nervous laughter]. I wish I didn't find out this way, but I am glad about that.

> **Tim Samson:** I feel that we go on hiking. I think I'm using my body, and I'm not using my body for anything that could possibly be sexualized love this [spring] time of year. I can feel that way when I get like really vigorous exercise. Some of it is probably endorphins…And there is like, there's a freedom. And I have some ability [to engage in running] that is very freeing, and I have the privilege of time to do that. And like and I, maybe it's as simple as this, it feels good. I like it. When I get to do things that feel good and I like them, that is pretty free…. Yeah, and…

> **Nichole:** (long pause) I think I'm at a point where I feel almost entirely free from (pause) sexual trauma. I think of it, it feels very distant to me, and I no longer operate on its terms. I like, think about it sometimes about like something that happened to me. I don't assume that all of my sexual partners are going to or like I don't assume that my roommates are going to harm me in some way or something like that. I don't regard people with suspicion. It's like, I'm not naturally feeling suspicion toward people that way.

Furthermore, Tim Samson's artwork, a poem speaking to the journey following sexual trauma, describes *internal relief* as an internal freedom with self-awareness; it partly reads as follows:

> *Leaning into trauma has a ring of freedom to it – and boy do I feel free these days. I'm not done, but the scared little boy*
> *Who centered himself to feel safe*
> *Is learning to sit with himself and be okay occasionally.*

These participant experiences of *internal relief* indicated that the **moments of relief** were associated with internal peace and freedom from the sexual violence. Participants also indicated the shift they noticed, emotionally, somatically, and psychologically, when they found reasons to hope that there was evidence of healing from sexual trauma. These internal moments of relief, specifically for Nathan, were related to his self-worth and awareness that he's likeable and attractive to those in the dominant group.

External relief. This second *subcategory* under the **moments of relief** refers to participants' experiences engaging with individuals and communities in their immediate social environment that contributed to moments of internal peace and freedom from systemic oppression. Some of these moments of *external relief* were experienced by participants collectively with others who share similar minority identities, as well as individually as participants experienced validation and acceptance from others. The *subcategory* of *external relief* was supported by properties of *interpersonal relational relief* and *societal relief.*

Interpersonal relational relief. This *property* is defined as moments of relief experienced by participants as a result of their interpersonal relationships with others closest to them. These interpersonal relationships are sources of validation and acceptance as well as of social support for the participants:

> **Tim Samson:** Yeah, I can feel it [moment of relief] when I interact with people [peers], like people that who's most of their focus, not their personality necessarily, but like their focus and their sort of hopes and dreams for themselves, is to be of help and to work on themselves and improve and be kind. It's really freeing to be around people that share my values.
>
> **Nichole:** I mean, there are other things that affect how I meet or interact with white men. (laughs) But and other than that, like I don't. I don't assume that all of my sexual partners are going to, or like I don't assume that my roommates are going to harm me in some way. or something like that. I don't regard people with suspicion. It's like, I'm not naturally feeling suspicion toward people that way.

Christina: ... I feel like one of the people who was able to support me more... she is also she's half Filipino and pansexual, and so I was able to talk to her a little bit more, not only about like my trauma, but the other things that were happening in my life. And since I felt more supported in those other areas because she was able to relate. And when she talked to me about what had happened to me. I knew, like it wasn't coming from a very outsidery perspective, if that makes sense. So even though she wasn't physically around, and I didn't get to talk to her as much, she was still, like, very foundational in the support. Just because of her, I guess, knowledge. So, I think it's not only within healthcare settings that we see this systemic, (pause) basically black and white way of thinking. But even without realizing it, like our friends and family will have that way of thinking, too.

River: ...one of my good friends recently, he said something, and I was like 'you know, so hang out with him [the aggressor] anymore?' And my friend was like "No, I might see him once a year or something", and then like I told him, and my friend was just like "oh, well, I won't be seeing him once a year anymore." 'No? Well, thank you. I appreciate that.'

Nathan: I think one thing another thing that's very freeing is being in an interracial relationship because my, my partner is white and she's very open to all of my Asian, all of my Asian heritage. She even cooked me some of my favorite dishes, like some of my favorite Asian dishes, which is very nice of her, and when I'll be like 'I don't think that this this tastes quite right. I think you might get a little more soy sauce, or a little of sugar or something' she'll be like "oh, okay, I didn't know I was just following the recipe", but it it's nice to see her so actively intertwined with my life in my culture, in that sense, and knowing that she wants to be a part of my life and wants to wants to promote that lifestyle...I know ,recently, we've talked about, you know, having kids or potentially someday having it. And I know one thing that we've talked about is we really want to make sure they're proud to be Asian, and they're proud to be a part of that cultural heritage. and I know that we'll probably use certain language. when teaching our kids like, I always called my Lola. Lola, which is like on my dad's side, Lola's grandmother, like we always use those words.. and I know that my mom, who's white, she always adapted like saying "anak" to me which is "son" to call me on a crowded place, and I'm glad that we can bridge cultures in that sense, and I'm glad that when we do enlighten people about certain races, they can kind of intertwine in a way that's that the unites the world, I guess. I am aware, however, that some people aren't fond of that that that kind of. But you know, I personally am because I come from a mixed household.

Societal relief. This second *property* under the *interpersonal relational relief* refers to participants' moments of relief from systemic oppression experienced collectively with others who also identify as having a minority status. In sharing the moments of *societal relief,* participants expressed moments of empowerment as they observed and interacted with those in positions of power such as professional experts who were able to normalize minority experiences. Participants identified specific moments where they were able to have relief from systemic oppression through their interactions in society:

> **Christina:** Um...there's been two times I felt, I guess, a little bit of relief [from systemic oppression]. And it was because I actually felt that my provider understood where I was coming from. That was my, she's my general practitioner here in [the States]. She is gay, and so, I went in, and I was like 'Hi!' I come from a non-supportive, I hadn't entirely told my family that, so I was like 'I come from a non-supportive family...' she was like "hey, are you pregnant now?" I was like 'no', you know, "you just told me you were active", and I was like 'I don't like men.' "Oh, okay, that's totally great. I have a wife." and I was like 'Nice! good for you' and then she just went about it like it was the most normal thing to have a partner of the same gender...and then just was telling me about everything that I needed to know that I probably wasn't told, and I wasn't, you know, to be safe to have a healthy relationship to check in on each other. Things that I probably wouldn't have been exposed to through another care provider. And then actually feel comfortable going to the doctor and not be, and not having them as like, 'oh, are you active?'. 'Yes.' 'Are you pregnant?' 'No.' 'What?' "What do you mean?" I mean "there's always a chance if you're active like..." 'No, there's not.' And so having that like actually makes me feel okay.

> **Christina:** Going to the doctor like I feel comfortable going and talking to her about like 'oh, us like I had the, TMI. I had a partner find like a little, I guess it was just inflamed, we found out, but an inflammatory portion. Of, me!' And so I went to my doctor, and I was like "Hi! worry and bodily thing.' And she's like, 'How do you know?' And I was like 'actually my partner.' And she was like "good on your partner. Okay, let's deal with this now." I was like 'thank you for not like thank you for just not making it a big deal for not... Just wanting to know how to make sure that it was like all safe but or being like understanding the situation.' And so that was, it was helpful. It was very helpful. And I like I haven't had that before.

> **Christina:** and then the second time was I had a therapist, and with many therapists I've had, both like just in general, if I go to a therapist, see if I like them, I found that it wasn't really, culturally, um, we didn't see eye to eye, culturally. So, I would be like 'here's my situation with my mom, who's brown', and they're like "talk back." And I was like 'no! (laughter) I prefer to live, thank you very much.' Like, I know I'm not going to talk back to my mom. So I had a therapist who was also a person of color, and so um, I was like 'this is my situation' and she was like 'oh, I know how that feels. You can't say anything now, can you?" and I was like 'No!'. 'you get it!' ...so, having that validation like culturally, and then having a validation through my sexual orientation by two care providers, it made me want to go back and talk to them. And made me want to, for therapy, go through my trauma, work through that, try to find solutions,

Nathan: to add to what kind of helped me heal, though, is there was a professor at my first semester who taught Asian American literature, and he was an Asian guy. He's really cool and he was very positive towards all Asian Americans, no matter what part of Asia they were from, he had a literature he from all of them, and he talked a lot about Asian masculinity, and he talked a lot about like just what it is to be an Asian man, and it was inspiring, and that helped me reclaim like a lot of my things. All the insecurities brought on by her [the aggressor] helped me, because this Asian dude was very confident. It was really awesome. Made me realize 'hey, it's okay to just be confident about it. If you're competent and on it, people will respect that culture.'

Nichole: (pause) (laughs) I think I have. I... so this, no, okay, this might actually feel dated in the long run. But there's a there's a community open mic event called Word Dog. I don't know if you have heard of it but it's run by a small community like it has a sort of staff, but it's mostly run on passion, it's every Tuesday. They don't have a set location, and so they announce it like every Sunday or something. But it's an open mic. People will sign up. And (pause) whoever signs up gets to share poems or they do impromptu storytelling as well. And they published two issues on donations, so far...There's a section at the end of Word Dog where people get to like, make big announcements, or ask for help and [the leader] sets up that time by saying that community is our greatest resource. I feel so safe around that sort of environment. Like what I bring to the table is enough to support my community because we're all doing that. That feels fun. It's also like I never see more people smoking weed and having a good time than at Word Dog, that's awesome (laughter), and they have dogs there like everyone brings their dogs and they hang out. That feels, I wish that more of my life was like that.

River: ...and one of the biggest ones [moments of relief from systemic oppression] was when I actually left the South, and I got out of [Southern State]. so, you explore the rest of the country. It was interesting because I got to see how other people react to the situations [exploring their identities and speaking up]. And yeah, I noticed, like, especially when I went to like the West Coast for the first time. It was like. I noticed people like my age. They were like standing up for themselves. In ways that is that like I never knew really, that people could.

Sophie: I experienced more relief when I'm talking with young people like teenagers who are more confident in their (pause) orientation and identity (pause) than I was or have been so that feels like a really safe population to be around. And then, at the same time, you know, like pride festivals are coming up. And, and there's even a Tell Us Something event to...there's a story telling event (audio cuts out) that happen to kind of like kick off the Pride Festival and I'd like to go there to kind of connect with more of my community. And then certainly having, being in [rural State] and being Pro LGBTQ population so yeah, I would say, the relief is more specific to being around kids who seem just genuinely self-accepting is what allows you to feel more also self-accepting and hopeful.

Sophie also added that observing the younger generation become more "confident" about owning and expressing their identities has contributed to moments of *societal relief*. However, she also raised the sense of fear for herself and others, especially in moments of collective expression and celebration of identities:

> **Sophie:** (pause) yeah, I think it's [moments of relief from systemic oppression] twofold ...and now I constantly have a fear of getting shot, basically, just with the amount of shootings that happen in the US. And then certainly having, being in Montana and being Pro LGBTQ population. On one hand, it's nice to start to have the words for self-expression and self-advocacy. And, on the other hand, it brings more negative attention, and therefore more risk.

Overall, the **moments of relief** for participants were related to two different types of trauma participants experienced: sexual trauma versus systemic oppression. **Moments of relief** from sexual trauma were associated with *internal relief* by experiencing internal peace and freedom, thus informing participants that the negative impacts and pain caused by the sexual trauma were reduced. *External relief*, on the other hand, was related to **moments of relief** from systemic oppression. The **moments of relief** from systemic oppression are associated with the acceptance, validation, and freedom participants experienced when interacting with others in their immediate social settings. The *external relief* may emerge from the *interpersonal relational relief* involving friends and participants' significant others while the *societal relief* is connected with freedom of identity expression both by themselves and others with minority identities.

Emerging processes

After the second-round analyses, PROCESSES were identified that served a pivotal role in the journey of healing from sexual trauma. These PROCESSES emerged based on participants' disclosure of phenomena that occurred over time and/or as they created meaning from the sexual violence experience. Nine PROCESSES were identified as essential components within the journey of sexual trauma.

The first PROCESS was INTERNALIZING BLAME TO EXTERNALIZIING BLAME. This process became clearer following the second-round analyses as participants explicitly described the importance of externalizing blame, so they could positively transform their views of who they are as well as their perceived role leading up to or following the event of sexual violence. The second PROCESS that was revealed was EXPOSURE TO NEW AND INCLUSIVE CULTURES and it facilitated **trauma response** and *external relief*. In reference to this PROCESS, participants disclosed the importance of finding a community with progressive perspectives that empowers them as well as creates an opportunity to explore who they are. This PROCESS of EXPOSURE TO NEW AND INCLUSIVE CULTURES was related to positive and helpful *behavioral responses* to trauma as well as *social support* upon disclosure of identities and the experience of sexual violence.

The third PROCESS was the SHIFT IN UNDERSTANDING OF CONSENT. During the first-round analyses, this PROCESS was identified as a dimension of shift from questioning to formulating an understanding of consent under the subcategory of family culture and socialization within the sociocultural contexts category. Following the second-round analyses, the shift from questioning to formulating an understanding of consent dimension was renamed as a shift in understanding of consent and reconceptualized as a PROCESS.

The fourth PROCESS was RECOGNIZING SEXUAL ENCOUNTER AS VIOLENCE. This PROCESS was created after reconceptualizing and renaming the dimension of naming and normalizing that was identified during the first-round analyses under the *subcategory* of *psychological responses*. The naming, accepting and normalization of the sexual violence and trauma experience came after participants were able to shift their understanding of consent. As a result, the PROCESS of RECOGNIZING SEXUAL ENCOUNTER AS A VIOLENCE enabled participants to recognize **trauma responses** and intentionally work towards strategies that facilitate healing.

The fifth PROCESS was TRIGGERS THAT LEAD TO NEGATIVE TRAUMA RESPONSES. This PROCESS was comprised of participants' fear of anticipated triggers as well as the reconceptualization of a subcategory of the perpetrators' attempt to contact the survivor; this had previously been created under the perpetrator category during the first-round analyses.

The sixth PROCESS was TIME WITH INTENTIONAL EFFORT as a means to create a buffer between the sexual violence encounter and the negative trauma responses. The role of passage of time was also discussed in terms of positive changes as well as the rise of large-scale social justice movements contributing to the **moments of relief** felt by participants.

The seventh PROCESS was SAFETY WITHIN THE SOCIOCULTURAL CONTEXTS LEADS TO MOMENTS OF RELIEF. This PROCESS represents the participants' process of noticing safety within their **sociocultural contexts and socializations** that contributed to their experience of moments of relief.

The eighth PROCESS was SOCIOCULTURAL CONTEXTS AND SOCIALIZATION SHAPE POWER AND PRIVILEGE. This PROCESS refers to the connections of the **power and privileges** both participants and their aggressor held and how these **power and privileges** were shaped by the *identity socializations* learned from the sociocultural contexts and socialization factors. Participants discussed the learned, earned, and unearned power and privileges their aggressor held as well as the *emotional burden* of their encounter with systems because of their underrepresented identities.

The last PROCESS identified during this second-round analysis was the PROCESS that connects the POSITIVE OUTCOMES of DISCLOSURE LEAD TO MOMENTS OF RELIEF AND POSITIVE TRAUMA RESPONSE. Participants shared the significant role of social support following a disclosure that provided an opportunity to emphasize the positive sexual trauma responses.

Below is a description of the PROCESSES identified and reconceptualized during the second-round analyses.

Process of internalizing blame to externalizing blame

The PROCESS of INTERNALIZING BLAME TO EXTERNALIZIING BLAME was created as *psychological responses* to highlight participants' shift from blaming themselves for their perceived role leading up to and following the sexual violence, to externalizing the blame and directing it towards the aggressor and the culture that enabled the aggressor. This shift in participants' responses contributed to an intentional focus on healing strategies rather than getting trapped in the negative **trauma responses**. Specifically, participants talked about the shift in externalizing shame and embarrassment as a significantly helpful process in their journey:

> River: So, I feel, I don't know, I'm just like really strong in my, like want to like, because I'm not embarrassed about it [sexual trauma] because there is nothing to be embarrassed about. I didn't do anything like the thing happened to me. It was really shitty. That's not my fault. So, I don't have. I don't have shame about it [shaking voice] which allows me to be open and talk to people and be like 'hey, just because you outwardly didn't say "No" it doesn't mean it was a "yes" ...and being like 'this was a

part of my life, still is obviously' but I could still separate it from myself. So, I don't know. It's been freeing in a way.

Tim Samson: when I when I think about how far I've come and how much I recovered from that like, it's a loosening of shame. But it's not like a happy feeling. It's like a "Yeah, that's not dogging me so much anymore. That's not like really making me like, it's not ruining my day."

Participants also shared the contributing factors that helped them to externalize the shame so they could experience slow but definite internal moments of relief from sexual trauma. Christina specifically talked about the importance of disclosure and social support in helping her ease the shame and transition to self-empowerment:

Christina: as I made new relationships and new friendships and had my support group that being like my friends, it was easier to talk about, easier to process, easier to kinda understand what had happened, and basically not put fault on myself.

For Tim Samson on the other hand, the shift to externalizing blame was related to getting answers about why and how the sexual trauma happened to him:

Tim Samson: there is something lovely about getting it like I get why this happens, and I know what my role in that, and I feel some shame around that. And I can sort of think about 'why do I feel shame?' And 'I cannot feel shame that I feel shame,' you know.

The self-empowerment of recognizing one's self-worth and value as a human being was also associated with externalizing blame for Nichole:

Nichole: …the connection it has to what your, your study is about specifically is like (long pause) like, I don't need to prove that I didn't deserve it, what happened to me. (laughs) In no way shape or form is that like something… Yeah. It's just, at least in my mind, it's like a fact that, yeah, none of that I deserved, and none of that (pause) was my fault.

Similarly, River reflected on the shift from INTERNALIZING THE BLAME TO EXTERNALIZING BLAME in her essay submitted as an artifact for this study. In this entry, River highlighted the importance of recognizing resiliency skills and persistence in order to externalize self-blame:

> *Eighteen years later I can finally say; Yes, I was a slut in my youth. Yes, I enjoy sex. Yes, [the aggressor] raped me. I have no shame because there's nothing to feel shame about. He didn't destroy me, I'm thriving! My only hope is that others can learn to regain their power, just like I did, and live in their truth. Because most of the time, all we have is the truth and our experiences.*

Participants' ability to shift from self-blame regarding their perceived contribution to the events that led to the sexual violence and/or their understanding of context, to externalizing the blame onto the aggressor or the existing culture that contributed to the encounter, was helpful in their trauma recovery. This shift to externalizing blame has helped to reduce the weight of the pain imposed on the participants by the sexual trauma.

Exposure to new and inclusive cultures

EXPOSURE TO NEW AND INCLUSIVE CULTURES refers to participants' efforts to change their social environment in search of a new setting that allows them to explore their identities and authentically present as they interact with others. The EXPOSURE TO NEW AND INCLUSIVE CULTURES sometimes involved changing their physical location and moving to a new community to find support and relief from the systemic encounters detrimental to their authentic existence.

River, for instance, talked about the pivotal role that moving out of her culture of origin had in helping her find her voice and experience more freedom to explore her identities:

> **River:** …one of the biggest ones [moments of relief from systemic oppression] was like when I actually left the South, and I got out of [southern State]. And I was like explore the rest of the country. It was interesting because I got to see how other people react to the situations. And I realized that Southern culture is very messed up in a lot of ways [laughter], and for a lot of part, especially women in the South are taught to just shut up and take it for a lack of better [words].

For River, this change to a more progressive, inclusive and tolerant culture was associated with learning more about the power of her voice. This effort to expose herself to other cultures helped River to find her voice and start to question and speak out against cultural norms that encouraged the silencing of women's voices. This assertive change was noticed by herself and others when she went back to her home state in the southern United States:

> **River**: Yeah. And then, like, when I did go back to the South, I was like, my, a lot of friends are like "Okay, damn, you're a lot more outspoken now" I'm like 'yes, because I know I can be.' It's like 'because I'm not getting shamed every time I speak up. And now I'm not afraid to get shamed [laughter] when I speak up.' So yeah, that was really important for me. It was just like getting out away from that ['do not make people uncomfortable'] mindset, and then I'm seeing other people, especially people that are like younger than me already, like able to stand up for themselves. And I'm like 'Oh, that's badass. I can do that like…' so which is really important, is like a 19-year-old… [silence] I feel like location is a big part of it.

Location was also important in how Christina was able to process a sexual violence experience that happened while attending university. The public health policies and guidelines that led to lockdowns and reintegration following COVID-19, moving back to her parents' home, and then coming back to the university where the sexual violence happened contributed to the prolonged trauma reactions:

> **Christina**: Mhmm. Yeah, yeah. So, I don't think I healed from what had happened to me in February [third sexual violence event] until after I had gone back to the university. Then like, basically that August so like it had taken me a full year of just being like 'I'll deal with that later, I'll deal with that later.' And then, when I was processing it, it felt like it was actually like right then and there. It was February again. I was…this is… it sucks.

The place where the sexual violence occurred was also related to the reminders and trigger. Christina shared the unavoidable encounters she had with location where the sexual violence happened because she had to be in that space once the COVID-19 lockdown policies were lifted. This pushed Christina to focus on "healing" from trauma and to no longer postpone processing it:

> **Christina**: So, I lived in the same hallway, just across from the room that I had my freshman year with where the situation had happened, and I had to stay in that. I was an RA for that hallway the following year. And I was like, 'Oh, okay, well, this is

going to be fun. I have to heal quick," or basically felt like I had to almost hurry my process because I didn't have the time during Covid, because I was focused on Covid and Black Lives Matter and being at home.

Moreover, Nichole shared the importance of moving to a new place associated with finding Yoga as a healing practice, and forming new and supportive social connections that contributed to positive body image and healing:

> **Nichole**: (long pause) That's a great question. (laughs) (pause) I wonder if I'm thinking of it as like um (pause) there are things that, like, like place was important for such [moment of relief] reasons, and trying to think of like what, aspects of this [healing] didn't necessarily have to do with place for me.
>
> **Nichole**: Yeah, I um, (pause)I have a lot of of independence here. And really do think that through the cohort and through other my other communities in [rural town], like have a chosen family (pause) that I felt safe talking to about these things. I don't know if that would have been true if I was living with my actual family. I also moved out of that house. Um, and I think part of the processing was setting up my new space. That felt really important. For sure.

Similarly, for Tim Samson, changing the social group and exposure to a social network that aligns with his values and goals have both been helpful in experiencing moments of relief:

> **Tim Samson**: Yeah, I can feel it when I interact with people in [peers], like people that who's most of their focus, not their personality necessarily, but like their focus and their sort of hopes and dreams for themselves, is to be of help and to work on themselves and like, improve and be kind like it's really freeing to be around people that share my values.
>
> **Tim Samson**: ahmm...and having a community of people who like want me to do that, you know, do that work. It's really like one of the artifacts of the patriarchy for me is that I have a hard time looking for help like I'll go to therapy, but like that's the therapy space, like in my social spaces, I have a hard time being like 'I'm having a hard time'... and just having people around me who are like "looks like you need some help" 'I think I do' is really, it's nice to be held accountable in a loving, caring sort of way like that. It's the first one I ever had. I kind of don't know what to do with it. It's such an abundance. I could call ten people right now, and I know they would pick up, and I know they would care even though we might not be like best friends, get together every day, it's like these are people that I have emotional connections with. I trust them. They trust me. We don't care that we're not perfect.

In summary, EXPOSURE TO NEW AND INCLUSIVE CULTURES was reported by participants as an important component in providing safety as well as perspectives that promoted relative freedom. This included the freedom to speak out and question the sociocultural factors that hinder participants' ability to explore their identities and process their traumatic experience. This PROCESS contributed to changing participants' views of the world and themselves, and to encouraging them to focus on healing from traumatic experiences.

Process of the shift in understanding of consent

The PROCESS of SHIFT IN UNDERSTANDING OF CONSENT was reconceptualized from a dimension of shift from questioning to formulating an understanding of consent during the first-round analyses, to become a PROCESS that connected the sexual violence incident with the RECOGNITION OF SEXUAL ENCOUNTER AS VIOLENCE. Specifically, during the second-round interview, participants discussed the shift in their understanding of the meaning of consent in a queer community. River, who disclosed the sexual trauma experience with her parents, reiterated the changes in how consent is defined now compared to her parents' generation:

> **River:** I'm like it was the seventies then, like you don't. You didn't know, you know, you really weren't told what you were supposed to do. Yeah, when you weren't told to stop your friends, you know?

Social justice movements played a significant role in making these disclosures possible and helping survivors to gain a new understanding of the meaning of consent. River noted the following in her artwork:

> *I never knew why this experience was so much grosser to me than any of the others, until 2017 and the #MeToo movement popped up. Rape was being redefined, or at least "defined." Then it all clicked. Steven raped me. I wanted to leave, I wanted to say no, I felt manipulated and like my life would get worse if I said no. Nothing got*

better though, he still tried his best to mock me at parties and try to keep my friends away from me. I felt like a plague. But it wasn't me, I'm not the problem. Sure, I liked to sleep around when single and when I chose to. Steven wasn't a choice, he never would've been a choice. He knew that, of course, he knew that.

Both Christina and Nichole shared the lack of inclusivity when consent is discussed, both in school and in communities, that leads individuals in the queer community to have less clarity to name and acknowledge sexual violence when it occurs. Christina shared the shift in her understanding of sexual violence in queer relationships following disclosure, which in turn had delayed her decision to share the experience with her family:

Christina: (long pause) This is gonna sound funny. At first, I didn't know that I had a trauma. And part of that was because...I mean I'd always heard about consent, and the very like straight way. I guess when you talk about consent, when you talk about sex and school, in whichever area, isn't used to talking or being inclusive to queer community, they're going to be very focused on the heterosexuality of it. And with that I didn't really, I didn't... I didn't really know. I knew that I had said, 'no', but I also was like 'well, this isn't what I learned' basically. Like my, my initial reaction was 'no, that, not that didn't happen to me because it wasn't a guy. It wasn't like, it wasn't basically what I had learned. It wasn't what I was taught', so I didn't realize that at first, but I knew that like I had this terrible feeling sitting in me,

Christina: and then it wasn't until after I talked to someone, they were straight, but like, I verbally expressed. And I was like 'yeah, this happened to me.' And they're like "are you okay? That was assault." That would- that was, "that's traumatic. Are you okay?" 'Oh, yeah, that. Yeah.' Now that I'm actually looking at the facts and taking gender out of everything, that was assault. I didn't fully realize it at first, because I had the idea of gender very stuck with me.

Christina: Oh, it took me a minute to realize it. Then, well don't talk about it [family culture on talking about negative emotions and experiences]. It almost had me feel like because I didn't realize it first and talk about it with like, at least my friends, how would I be able to, like, then speak about it to my family? I don't know if that makes sense.

Nichole also shared their pre-trauma understanding of consensual sexual encounters especially as a queer and, due to the experience with sexual violence, the shift after the sexual trauma:

> **Nichole**: Hmm. yeah, interesting. (long pause) There's this... there's a book called *In the Dream House* by Carmen Maria Machado, which is about intimate partner violence in queer relationships, and how, at least in a in queer affirming communities, we like, we sort of like to think of queer relationships as somehow pure or more safe. Or like more whatever it is than cis-het ones. But, like sexual violence occurs among queer people, too.
>
> **Nichole**: And so, I thought to myself, like (pause) the, I guess maybe, I'm like freshly processing this, but it's possible that, like, I had this assumption that being queer would protect me from the things like (pause) from those things that I hear about all the time, because I never hear about them in queer relationships.

Similar to Christina, Nichole noted the lack of language and open communication related to sexual violence and abuse in relationships in the queer community, especially when it involves individuals who identify as non-binary:

> **Nichole**: *Come and Bring Him Into the Shadows* book is like describes this Lesbian couple where one of them was deeply abusive, but no one really knew, and, in fact, sometimes lesbian couples are able to mask all that really well. So anyway, that's what [is] coming to mind first. Um (pauses) it also feels, um, I don't know if people have a good way of talking about... (pause) I... like a specific way of talking about sexual violence toward non-binary people, because it has so much to do with like genitals. (laughs)

Overall, the SHIFT IN UNDERSTANDING OF CONSENT has been a significant part of the journey following sexual trauma. Participants in the queer community specifically talked about the lack of knowledge, language, and normalizing of consent within queer relationships. Participants' process of SHIFT IN UNDERSTANDING OF CONSENT was facilitated by disclosure of sexual violence and/or acquiring knowledge about queer relationships so participants could name and normalize the sexual trauma. Social justice movements such as the MeToo movement also contributed to this SHIFT IN UNDERSTANDING OF CONSENT.

Recognition of sexual encounter as violence

The dimension of naming and normalizing that was under the *psychological responses* to trauma was reconceptualized as a PROCESS of RECOGNITION OF SEXUAL ENCOUNTER AS VIOLENCE. This PROCESS refers to participants' journey of acknowledging the sexual encounter with their aggressor as a violation, and then starting to recognize their reactions to the sexual encounter as a violation and/or traumatic. This process of RECOGNITION OF SEXUAL ENCOUNTER AS VIOLENCE can be best facilitated by the SHIFT IN UNDERSTANDING OF CONSENT. For instance, River wrote in her essay about the power of naming and recognizing the sexual encounter as violence:

> *Once I could name it, I could box it up and put it on a shelf. It could live outside my body and I could finally tell it to people in a way it made sense.*

Both Christina and Tim Samson also shared their process of recognizing what happened to them as sexual violence. For Christina, this meant reconceptualizing the role of gendered constructs in relationships, while Tim Samson needed to gain more understating of the role of patriarchy and workplace culture. Both of them mentioned the role of support from others in naming the sexual encounter as violent and traumatic before they were able to recognize it as such:

> **Christina:** like, I verbally expressed. And I was like, 'yeah, this happened to me.' And they're like "are you? Okay? That was assault. That was, that's traumatic. Are you? Okay?" 'Oh, yeah, that!' Now that I'm actually looking at the facts and taking gender out of everything. That was a, I didn't fully realize it at first, because I had the idea of gender very like stuck with me.
>
> **Tim Samson:** ahm…And so really, it wasn't until like, I mentioned this before, like 10 years later, that I was talking about it [sexual violence] with a therapist, and just sort of like, "I'm going to stop you because I'm pretty sure that you got sexually assaulted quite a bit." And so, just been, in revisiting that, it's interesting how much like the, and this is what lot of this comes out in the poem, how I, um, I'm angry that people treated my body as though it wasn't mine. but more than anything, just that time, for, like nothing was mine, like everything was just on a conveyor belt that somebody else is

pushing the button and I didn't realize, even though I followed my dreams, and, like I, I ostensibly chose to do this career in retrospect.

As a result, the process of RECOGNITION OF SEXUAL ENCOUNTER AS VIOLENCE was stated as one of the major components as survivors navigate the journey following sexual violence. Once they were able to name and recognize sexual violence, it was possible for participants to start recognizing their responses to trauma and its triggers as well as notice the moments of relief.

Time with intentional effort

The PROCESS of TIME WITH INTENTIONAL EFFORT emerged during the second-round analyses. Participants discussed the role of time in two ways: the passage of time that involved rising social justice movements and awareness of the diversity of identities, and the everyday time filled with intentional effort to recover from trauma. For instance, Tim Samson shared the importance of intentional effort to process trauma as time passes, stating that the passage of time by itself was not helpful to the journey of trauma recovery:

> **Tim samson**: There are days where I'm just like I feel so free. I feel so great. And there are days I'm like I'm so aware of my appearance. I'm so aware of my body in ways I know we're super informed by this time of my life [time of sexual violence]. All within the span of a week. So, like in some ways, it's like this, Whoop! Whoop! Whoop! Whoop! um in terms of time. Certainly. So, I think time in a vacuum, I would have learned to forget about it, and it would have been this thing that was just hanging out, probably bothering me in subconscious ways. Time plus active work, therapy education, like intentionality, has been tremendous because I don't, it's not so close anymore that I that it is untouchable, but it's not yet so far away that it's unrememberable. I can really be in this sort of lovely safe place…and, like time is necessary for me to be able to get to that place, but I think time by itself was insufficient.

Nathan also shared the importance of engaging himself in activities that felt productive and fulfilling as time passes and ones that help to create meaning out of the sexual trauma he encountered:

Nathan: Another thing that I've done with time, um, in regards to time is I think, that filling your time with activities or hobbies or personal goals helps you overcome thinking about negative things especially when you have spiraling thoughts that kind of lead back to one thing and like, whenever I'm about to go into those, those downward spirals of thoughts, I always feel it's best to just not think about it and do something else like a different activity. So, I've taken up a lot of hobbies too.

Nathan: Time itself plays a role in how, how you develop, but I also think that in order for you to develop and move past certain things, you need to have different experiences that help you see different perspectives. And I feel like my more positive experiences have come from my hobbies. I play a lot more music. I do a lot more physical activity. I see a therapist now, like feeling my time with all these different things really helps me just get better and better and better. And I feel like that being in a schedule, a routine, that is also really important. Just on a personal level, like it might be different for someone else. But for me

Participants also shared the relevance of time in creating a buffer between the sexual violence event and the intense negative trauma responses by intentionally delegating time to process emotional responses. Nichole, for example, stated that they deliberately shifted their attention and focus to work and other life events immediately after the sexual violence incident, giving them an opportunity to be intentional in allotting time and space to process the trauma:

Nichole: …what aspect of the healing are more time based? Um, I think the way that I described things needed to be, when it happens, (pause) and it wasn't the most truthful representation of what happened. But I couldn't expect myself to understand it right away. And I knew that. And I was 'this feels really bad right now', and I know that, like the way I'm talking about myself and other people about this isn't super honest, but I just need to like go to work, (laughs) and I need to go to class, and I think I'll have bandwidth for this processing (pause) over time, but I can't do it all right now. I think that was something like, so I'm not someone who needs to be convinced to do my emotional processing, and so it's not like I was putting it off on purpose or avoiding it, but I knew that (pause) I would naturally give myself time for it. What I, but I was more worried that I would allow the feeling of the processing to overtake, um, my other responsibilities. So, I just sort of needed to flatten the curve of it all.

In one instance, Christina noted the impact of the Covid-19 pandemic and associated public health guidelines that forced everyone to limit social interactions and simultaneously minimized the social support that existed before the pandemic. Christina also shared that emerging family issues during Covid-19 took priority because, while living with her family, she could get more support for family matters. This delayed the intentional focus on creating meaning from sexual trauma and engaging in healing practices:

> **Christina**: And then I went home to a not so fun situation back home. And my support group was now all online because they were everyone was back home. So it was like, well, even if I wanted to stay in [Western State], it wasn't like I would be able to still have them there, so that I think slow down my healing process because I wasn't just trying to heal from what had happened in February, but I was trying to deal with my situation in the moment.

> **Christina**: Yeah, no one knew what to do. And during that half year I also, I didn't know what to do, and I didn't know how to heal. During that time, too, I was. It was a lot of things happening during that time. So, it I feel like when you try to pile on things to process the things to heal from something that happened before COVID was gonna get like pushed back.... I don't have the support for that right now. But I have the support for this. So, I'm going to focus on this because I can... I can work on that. So, I think, COVID it just... it really, it messed with like the sense of time, but also just the healing process. And (pause) how, I think, had COVID not happened, I would have healed a lot quicker, yeah, it was it (long pause) hard. Yeah. It was because it took me longer to heal.

While most participants talked about time in terms of their engagement in intentional trauma recovery and healing activities, River emphasized the role time had played especially when it came to getting some relief from systemic oppression:

> **River**: yeah, a lot, actually, time is, I feel like time is extremely important. um... I mean, because I mean for one, it took me a long time to actually figure out that what I went through was, you know, a sexual trauma, and not just like a drunk one-night stand, which is, you know, what I thought of it as a long time, which is why I like. When I figured out what it was, I was like 'no, I am just being dramatic', but like with time. I realized one 'No, I wasn't being dramatic'. And two 'yes, it was a thing that happened to me. It was it just a drink one night', and so time is just giving me, like a good perspective to just like actually name it and then process it, and now, separated it from myself which is probably not something I could have done it like [at]18 or 20 [years old].

Here is what River noted on her art submission:

> *Time has given me perspective. I'm able to name it, call it what it was, and tell others that their stories are valid. Rape and sexual assault can happen in many forms, in many ways. It's not black and white, in fact, the gray area is probably where it*

happens the most. It's not my fault, any of it. It's not my fault for drinking or going to parties or even staying. Steven was the one who made the choice to rape me, to not let me leave, to dangle my friendships in front of me. But I named it, and in doing that, I reclaimed the power I had lost to him. He's not a bully that holds any power. He's pathetic and disgusting.

Sophie shared her thoughts on time and negative **trauma responses** in which the response to sexual trauma is non-constant:

Sophie: (pause) I guess one thing that I'm thinking about is that it's not, like the suffering from the trauma is not constant. So, there's, and that's, I guess, one of the nice distinctions, too, between like complex childhood trauma versus PTSD, where ideally, it's only coming up when I have that trigger versus just being constant.

On the other hand, Sophie indicated that time does not really have an important role in recovering from trauma:

Sophie: Uhh…(pause) I think that's the frustrating part, that it doesn't feel like it [time] (pause) is playing the role that (pause) this idea that time heals all, I think, is less applicable when you have a trauma disorder, right? That you're still, you're still living in it now. And so, the amount of time between now and whenever something happened is kind of irrelevant if your body is still telling you that it's happening now.

In summary, participants reported that trauma recovery and healing are associated with their PROCESS of TIME WITH INTENTIONAL EFFORT. They also emphasized the role of intentional and active engagement in activities, hobbies and decisions that allow them to explore the meaning of sexual trauma.

Triggers lead to negative somatic and emotional responses of trauma

This PROCESS of TRIGGERS LEAD TO NEGATIVE SOMATIC AND EMOTIONAL RESPONSES OF TRAUMA was partly a reconceptualization of the *perpetrator's attempt to contact the survivor*, a subcategory under **the perpetrator** during the first-round analyses. This process refers to the ongoing nature of events and/or trauma responses that reminded participants of the traumatic experience and shadowed the positive lights obtained by the moments of relief.

Sophie explained the occurrence of trauma symptoms as intermittent, happening upon the experience of a triggering circumstance:

> **Sophie:** I guess, one of the nice distinctions, too, between like complex childhood trauma versus PTSD, where ideally, it's only coming up when I have that trigger versus just being constant.

> **Sophie:** I guess in this moment it feel it kind of represents frustration that I feel, like, I have that even with growth (pause) and personal development that [sexual trauma] (pause) history is still very much alive in me. And I haven't done therapy work specifically on that, and I would expect that to make a difference. But for now, it just keeps coming up, yeah, it's still present.

Nathan wrote, in his poem, the sadness he experienced especially after witnessing what he felt was a singular attention given to women sexual trauma survivors during the rising of the #MeToo Movement:

> *I started the semester off with it in the back of my mind. I tried not to, but somedays it was all I thought about. There was an assault march I got stuck in while heading to my poetry class. The participants held signs, waved flags, chanted how they believed survivors. Me too. But then I remembered that it can't happen to boys so I ran to the bathroom, cried, wore sunglasses so no one would see, thanked god the mask mandate covered the emotions on my face.*

To represent the ongoing nature of triggers and the difficulty in the healing of sexual trauma, Sophie shared a song by the Interrupters, *In the Mirror*, as part of the artwork to indicate her journey with sexual trauma:

> *No matter how far I run, I always end up back here*
> *No matter how far I go, I always end up back here*
> *Took me two years to write this song*
> *I wanted it perfect, no wrinkles in it*
> *Took me a long time to come clean*
> *To be honest, the truth's so ugly*
> *Took me a long time to come home*
> *I didn't think you'd get me*
> *I had too much explaining*

> *No matter how far I run, I always end up back here*
> *No matter how far I go, I always end up back here*
> *In the mirror, in the mirror, in the mirror, only in the mirror*
> *I always felt so out of place*
> *In a crowded room, I speak too soon, yeah*
> *I put a big smile on my face*
> *I can't let them know it's all for show, no*
> *Took me a long time to come home*
> *I didn't think you'd get me*
> *I had too much explaining*
> *No matter how far I run, I always end up back here*
> *No matter how far I go, I always end up back here*
> *In the mirror, in the mirror, in the mirror, only in the mirror*
> *I'm tired of running*
> *No matter how far I go, I always end up back here*
> *In the mirror, in the mirror, in the mirror, only in the mirror*

Sophie stated that triggers may not be directly related to sexual encounters, but rather could be associated with loss of a secure intimate relationship that serves as a reminder that there is more to be done to heal:

> **Sophie:** Um, I think what's interesting is that the breakup that I just went through like two months ago really impacts what piece of art I would have sent to you because I was just, I was hopeful that it meant that, like you know, my trauma, that I had enough corrective experiences that, because I-I was no longer experiencing like PTSD symptoms with my partner. But, um, but I was curious if that would really, that it was gone, or that I was securely attached to that person, and something that I've noticed right away, not related to, not related to sex or even physical intimacy, but it was just that, that break up has left me feeling just a lot less safe and secure in my own body, I think, cause I have a pretty anxious attachment style.

Moreover, Sophie highlighted her anticipation of experiencing trauma symptoms if she were to engage in physical intimacy in the future:

> **Sophie:** So, um, now going back to feeling less confident and less secure in my own body, which I think is true for a few reasons. I feel like it's... it would, it would be very fair for me to expect myself to have more reactions again, more like trauma reactions. should I be intimate with somebody in the future. And so, that song had this pattern of like this idea of like, I'm gaining insight, and I'm making headway, and no matter how much headway I see myself making, I still end up finding myself getting tripped up back in the same visceral space or head space.

Overall, participants shared the intermittent events that serve as triggers and sometimes related to the aggressor's attempt to contact them following the sexual violence encounter. In some cases, the TRIGGERS associated with NEGATIVE SOMATIC AND EMOTIONAL RESPONSES OF TRAUMA were anticipated patterns of behaviors that led to frustrations for the survivors.

Safety within the sociocultural contexts leads to moments of relief

This PROCESS of SAFETY WITHIN THE SOCIOCULTURAL CONTEXTS LEADS TO MOMENTS OF RELIEF refers to participants' journey of finding safety within their social, cultural, and contextual systems that allows them to experience moments of relief. Some of these safety moments were received from relationships with those that shared an identity, or with those with comparable power and privilege based on the sociocultural and contextual factors of the survivor. Christina, for instance, shared the sense of safety within the sociocultural setting that was related to continuous communications and connections with someone who shares similar power and privilege related to their intersecting identities. She explained the difference in quality of relationships and feelings of being understood based on the identity of the person in her social group:

> **Christina**: so a lot of my healing journey was being heard. But it was very few times where it was like I felt understood… So, I have to be understanding for myself if you come from a different culture, it's so hard to find that relatable relationship… I think like combining different I guess cultures, because I feel like if you're BIPOC, you have a culture. But there's also, like the LGBTQ queer gay culture. And so then, trying to combine those to support someone else's, it's funky if you're only a part of one or not a part of either… I think. when someone shares about their healing process to their or shares their situation to their support group to their friends, they're going to be supportive of the person, but it might be harder to take into account if they can't really [understand] the culture around it.

On the other hand, when the larger sociocultural contexts and socializing environments are not changing and not supportive of the journey of the survivor, the survivors' emotional burden increases as they must do all the work of healing without the changes in social and cultural contexts needed to facilitate healing. . Sophie specifically stated the survivor's emotional burden related to not having a clearly defined "functional environment" that could facilitate healing:

> Sophie: (pause) Umm. Well, I think that it means that the environment in which I need to heal in is going to stay the same. Probably throughout my lifetime. And because I think there's different ways to heal. There's, there's getting into a new, more functional environment. But that doesn't really feel like an option, (pause) as much as doing internal work to learn, umm, to trust myself and also learn that I can bounce back if something bad happens.

> Sophie: Right. I think it makes it, again, that the the...(pause). It's not a restorative justice model, by any means. So it feels like it's on the healer, um, to do the work. There is not really any kind of reparation. So it's I in that way? I guess it feels like a just a continued burden.

Similarly, Nichole shared that their healing journey from sexual trauma was focused on their feminine side because the sociocultural context and socializing allows for the feminine identity to easily have a conversation about what it means to have sexual trauma; this is in sharp contrast to trauma response exploration from a masculine perspective:

> Nichole: Like I did, I almost want. I felt more- I feel like I do still have some processing to do of the event. From, from a masculine place. If that makes sense. I have done, like more processing from a feminine posture like, I, uh (pause) because I am fem, (pause) maybe you feel like more... not pressure... But that's the this, really, um (pauses) it's the easier conversation to have… mhmm (pause). But the part of me that, like I, the part of me that experienced that as a masculine person also, like, I think, wants some room for that, yeah, (pauses) that's my thought. (laughs)

> Nichole: I felt more- I feel like I do still have some processing to do of the event, from a masculine place, if that makes sense. I have done, like more processing from a feminine posture like, I, uh (pause) because I am fem, (pause) maybe you feel like more... not pressure... But that's the this, really, um (pauses)…mhmm (pause). But the part of me that, like I, the part of me that experienced that as a masculine person also, like, I think, wants some room for that.

In this PROCESS of SAFETY WITHIN THE SOCIOCULTURAL CONTEXTS LEADS TO MOMENTS OF RELIEF, participants discussed the role of safe connections with those who share the same power and privilege as they have within their social contexts. Conversely, the lack of safety and social justice restoration within the larger community can lead to more pressure on the survivor to heal without comparable changes in the social environment.

Sociocultural contexts and socialization shape the power and privilege

Participants shared that the **power and privileges** that they themselves and their aggressor held were connected to their immediate as well as larger sociocultural contexts and socializing factors. The PROCESS that the **sociocultural contexts and socializations** that shaped the **power and privilege** the participants and their aggressor held were discussed in relation to the societal norms that inform who has power and who does not. For instance, Sophie shared the connection of norms around gender and power that gives men more power and privilege:

> **Sophie:** Oh, yeah. Yeah, absolutely. I think, you know, trauma or not, I think we're like taught to be (long audio cut off) But yeah, I definitely think that there is just an, um, inherent yeah, an inherent fear of men and the power...which is interesting [thinking] but but yeah, I guess I certainly do feel I would assume that even without the trauma there is this layer of, of fear, of the oppressive population, and part of that too, I think, is anatomy.
>
> **Sophie:** If the man was the...Oh, yeah, I think whether or not people, whether or not a female has trauma, I think we're still taught to be prepared to be attacked and that, like women can be raped by men, but not by other women.

These gendered power and privileges heightened the power men have and contributed to getting triggered during intimate relationships. Although Sophie was hesitant to definitively state the connection between gendered socializations and **power and privilege**, she identified the differences in her experience of triggers during initial intimacy with men versus women:

> **Sophie:** (long pause) Um, (pause) I would say that I definitely have more of a, (pause) I found myself to be a lot more, um, like triggered and like have, like panic attacks and hyperventilating when I'm initially intimate with men versus with women. And that is independent of any of their behavior. so definitely, I feel like it's hard to say if it's because I feel more accepted by another female or non-male person, or if it's because the trauma was with a male, so it's hard to pull those two pieces apart for sure. but that's where I would, you know, that's where I guess there's most notable, um, relief...mhmm

Moreover, River shared the role of her culture of origin in creating the general sense of fear to speak up against unwanted advances during or after the event. River shared that this sociocultural context has relation to the power of the aggressor:

> **River:** I noticed, like, especially when I went to like the West Coast for the first time...I noticed people like my age, they were like standing up for themselves in ways that Is that like I never knew really, that people could....part of the weird Southern culture of like, "Oh, don't make people uncomfortable." And I'm like, 'why?' So,it's like, maybe like question things and maybe like not afraid to like...because, like most of the time the people that you're not supposed to make uncomfortable usually the abusers.

Nathan also discussed the lesser **power and privilege** associated with racial minorities and the intersection of identifying as a man that leads to more fear and less power for him as an Asian American:

> **Nathan:** I think that [silence] I think that ethnic people are often considered scary to most white people. I mean, we we can talk about like yellow peril or like how White women being rape was often the thing of like the cost for a lot of lynching, you know, like these types of things happen. So I think that just being a white woman who who can kind of she has a certain value, social value, and it's different than than ethnic women. And please forgive me if that's ignorant because I could be completely wrong.

Therefore, having a strong ownership of one's own cultural and *racial identity* helps participants to protect themselves from the *emotional burden* associated with the encounter with the system and those with greater power and privilege:

> **Christina:** I think it's because I am very set, and being a proud Latin person, proud Mexican. So I don't let a lot of that waiver for me. I've had partners who are like you need to basically stop being so ethnic of like, stop celebrating your culture so much. And I'm like, no turn on Mariachi music and dance away. So what like, yeah, that's not

going to happen. I'm proud of who I am. so I'm going to stick with that. So I feel, in that route It was, I was okay.

In summary, in this PROCESS of the SOCIOCULTURAL CONTEXTS AND SOCIALIZATION SHAPE THE POWER AND PRIVILEGE. This influenced the identity based learned views, perspectives and values, and impacted how the participants' encounter with the system. The **power and privilege** learned from the **sociocultural contexts and socializations** and held by the aggressors has impacted the participants' trauma response especially in relation to triggers as participants continue their healing journey from sexual trauma.

Positive disclosure outcomes lead to moments of relief and positive trauma response

Participants revealed that the interpersonal outcomes of disclosures, specifically social support, were related to internal moments of relief:

> **Tim Samson:** and having a community of people who like want me to do that, you know, do that work. It's really like one of the artifacts of the patriarchy for me is that I have a hard time looking for help like I'll go to therapy but like that's the therapy space, like in my social spaces, I have a hard time being like 'I'm having a hard time' and just having people around me who are like "looks like you need some help" 'I think I do' is really... it's nice to be held accountable in a loving [and] caring sort of way like that.... It's such an abundance. I could call ten people right now, and I know they would pick up, and I know they would care even though we might not be like best friends, get together every day, these are people that I have emotional connections with I trust them. They trust me. We don't care that we're not perfect.
>
> **River:** ...one of my good friends recently, he said something, and I was like 'you know, so hang out with him [the aggressor] anymore? And my friend was like "No, I might see him once a year or something", and then like I told him, and my friend was just like "oh, well, I won't be seeing him once a year anymore." 'No? Well, thank you. I appreciate that.' He's like "I have no clue" but I'm like 'well, it's a long time to like figure it out, but I was like that. That's the thing' and he's like "I'm really afraid. Sorry." I'm like 'it's okay...[laughter] you [are] the good one' And it's like 'I don't blame you for being friends with them, because, like, you don't know.'
>
> **Christina:** A lot of my friends are straight and white, which I am not straight or white but half white, and so when I guess when they were supporting me, they were doing it in the best way that they could, but support groups don't always know how to be the

best if they can't relate. So even though they were very supportive, and they were very...they got me through everything. So that definitely was great. But I feel like one of the people who was able to support me more, she moved. how rude! But she is also she's half Filipino and so I was able to talk to her a little bit more, not only about like my trauma, but the other things that were happening in my life. And since I felt more supported in those other areas because she was able to relate. And when she talked to me about what had happened to me, I knew it wasn't coming from a very outsidery perspective if that makes sense. So even though she wasn't physically around, and I didn't get to talk to her as much, she was still, like, very foundational in the support. Just because of her, I guess, knowledge, we see this systemic basically black and white way of thinking. But even without realizing it, like our friends and family will have that way of thinking, too.

However, undesirable interpersonal outcomes of disclosure i.e., victim *questioning* was related to negative experiences in the trauma healing for participants. This was evident in participants' experiences of getting questioned which sometimes led to negative emotional responses to trauma:

> **Nichole:** Yeah, I remember like getting questions like, 'Okay, but what did you... how were you...' I was like, no, I don't want to answer these questions. (laughs) It's awful.

> **Nathan:** So I I think that when we think about sexual trauma or sexual assault towards men, or just sexual assault towards anyone in general, we we we usually give it more towards women or feminine identities. And I think that [silence] that's that's fair I think that women have it rougher than men do and even though it really hurts my feelings that no one most people probably don't care about me as much. I understand it. And it's something that I feel like I just need to get over.

River wrote the following in an essay showing her process of responding to getting questioned after disclosing her experience with sexual trauma:

> *Once I could name it, I could box it up and put it on a shelf. It could live outside my body and I could finally tell it to people in a way it made sense. Some friends were skeptical: "But like, he didn't have a gun to your head."*
> *I had to tell them; "just because he wasn't about to murder me doesn't mean it's not rape." Because I know there's a gray area that this situation falls into. If I was to stand up in front of a jury, he would never be convicted and I would be slut shamed. This is one reason why victims don't speak up, they don't think anything will come of it, especially not anything good. It doesn't matter how many people I chose to sleep with; before and after...those were choices. Steven wasn't a choice.*

In sum, the outcomes of disclosure have an impact on participants' reaction and journey following a sexual violence encounter. Often, *social support* leads participants to feel heard and provides a moment of relatable-ness and internal peace while *victim questioning* leads to negative *emotional responses* complicating the healing journey from sexual trauma.

Conclusions of second round analysis

Following the second-round analysis, five categories that portrayed the experience of healing from sexual trauma were identified. Participants discussed the **sociocultural contexts and socializations** that impacted their identity exploration and formation. They also shared the importance of family cultures and their upbringings as they formed their sense of self and established and maintained relationships. These **sociocultural contexts and socializations** fed into the **power and privilege** both they and their aggressor held within a shared social, cultural and contextual environment. Often the aggressor held greater power and privilege compared to the survivor with intersecting minority identities. The act of **disclosure** of the sexual violence and trauma to survivors' social relationships was accompanied by either social support that helped participants to feel heard and validated or victim questioning in which participants needed to justify the circumstances around consent during the sexual encounter. Once participants were able to name and recognize the sexual encounter as violence, they were able to be intentional in their strategies to recover from the trauma. **Trauma responses** to the sexual violence incorporated somatic, emotional, psychological and behavioral processes that were sometimes negative and other times connected to **moments of relief**. Participants shared that *internal relief* was related to healing from sexual trauma while *external relief* was mostly related to moments of freedom from the systemic oppression.

These five categories identified during the second-round analysis were facilitated by nine PROCESSES that assisted participants as they made meaning of the sexual trauma experience. The shift from INTERNALIZING BLAME TO EXTERNALIZIING BLAME contributed to participants' focus on positive trauma responses rather than the negative ones. Moreover, participants' conscious attempt to use TIME WITH INTENTIONAL EFFORT has helped them to be emotionally aware and focus on helpful **trauma responses**. However, to be intentional about the time and energy they were spending on healing, participants must experience a positive SHIFT IN UNDERSTANDING OF CONSENT and start to recognize that the sexual encounter happened without their consent. This was related to their process of RECOGNIZING SEXUAL ENCOUNTER AS VIOLENCE and naming themselves as survivors of sexual trauma. The process of naming and recognizing the sexual encounter as trauma was facilitated by the POSITIVE OUTCOMES of DISCLOSURE LEAD TO MOMENTS OF RELIEF AND POSITIVE TRAUMA RESPONSE. The EXPOSURE TO NEW AND INCLUSIVE CULTURES helped participants recognize the **sociocultural contexts and socializations** related to their place of origin and the **power and privilege** related to *identity socializations*. This exposure to new norms and cultures also helped participants focus on healing orientated **trauma responses**. The **trauma response and moments of relief** were shaped by the TRIGGERS participants encountered that lead to negative **trauma responses**.

CHAPTER 5: WEATHERING THE STORM: THE JOURNEY OF HEALING FROM SEXUAL TRAUMA

For this grounded theory study, I conducted twelve interviews with six survivors of sexual violence with the aim of developing a theory about the journey of healing from sexual trauma. These six survivors identified as members of an underrepresented group based on one or more of their identities in relation to race, sexual identity, gender identity, or disability identity. Through my engagement with these participants, I learned that the positionality and **power and privilege** they held in the world were shaped by the intersection of these underrepresented identities. Moreover, their aggressors held positions of greater **power and privilege** than did the participants prior to and during the event of the sexual violence. The **sociocultural contexts and socializations** in which the participants and their aggressors were situated played a significant role in the **power and privileges** and in the ways survivors reacted to their encounter with sexual trauma. The processes of the SHIFT IN UNDERSTANDING OF CONSENT and RECOGNIZING the SEXUAL ENCOUNTER AS VIOLENCE had major and substantial roles as survivors began to intentionally take steps towards healing and integrating sexual trauma into their journey.

Within the **trauma response**, the process of transitioning from INTERNALIZING BLAME TO EXTERNALIZING BLAME was significant for encouraging survivors' engagement in positive *behavioral responses* and *psychological responses.* These responses gradually outweighed the *somatic responses* and negative *emotional responses* such as *shame and guilt* associated with their sexual violence experience. As survivors continued to intentionally devote time and effort to healing, they were able to experience **moments of relief** characterized by an internal sense of peace and freedom, thus informing them that the pain caused by the sexual trauma was becoming less impactful in their lives. This journey of healing from sexual trauma and the moments of *internal relief* were connected to the *social support* survivors received upon disclosing their sexual trauma to significant others. However, negative *interpersonal outcomes of disclosure* like *victim questioning* contributed to *somatic* and *emotional responses* leading survivors to question their experience with sexual trauma.

The Boat

The theory of the journey of healing for survivors of sexual trauma is depicted as a boat (see Figure 6) sailing on water. The boat represents the healing journey as survivors stay afloat and devote their energy to healing following an encounter with sexual violence. The boat represents the five categories identified in this study, **sociocultural contexts and socializations, power and privilege, trauma response, disclosure** and **moments of relief,** and how they relate to each other as survivors give meaning to their traumatic experience and integrate it into their lives.

The boat is constructed from planks of wood representing the PROCESSES significant in connecting the **trauma responses** with the changes in perspectives and actions that enabled survivors to intentionally work on trauma healing strategies. These PROCESSES were facilitated by **disclosures** and the *social support* that followed the disclosure of the sexual trauma, while the *undesirable outcome of disclosure* (*victim blaming*) created stagnation in the healing journey. **Disclosure** either happened immediately following the sexual violence encounter and/or during and after survivors began their engagement with healing-focused trauma responses.

The boat's wheel represents the **trauma response** cycle that is filled with immediate to ongoing *somatic responses* and *emotional responses* that ranged from *emotional* *awareness* to *shame and guilt* and then a shift from <u>anger</u> to righteous anger. The **trauma responses** also consist of *behavioral responses* through which survivors sought to develop helping strategies, so that the cycle of negative *somatic responses* and *emotional responses* did not overshadow the healing strategies. Combined with a positive shift in the *psychological responses*, the *behavioral responses* of trauma helped survivors steer the wheel toward integrating trauma into their journey. Moreover, the sail of the boat represents the **moments of relief**, both external and internal, that help the boat stay afloat and continue moving forward in their healing journey. The weather surrounding the boat is not always smooth, comfortable, and peaceful, but rather the boat keeps floating under a cloud of potential triggers that may appear at any point. These triggers were survivors' encounters with reminders of the sexual trauma experience, eliciting restored negative *somatic responses* and *emotional responses*. These triggers could also be associated with the continued *emotional burden* survivors experienced due to their <u>encounter with the system</u>. Although **trauma response** begins following an incident of sexual violence, it continues through the ongoing and intentional recognition of trauma reactions and the integration of healing strategies, which were connected to how survivors perceived and interpreted their **sociocultural context and socializations** as well as the **power and privileges** both the survivor and their aggressor held.

The water underneath the boat represents these **sociocultural contexts and socialization** that contribute to the survivors' *identity socialization*. These *identity socializations* are influenced by the *family culture and upbringings* that survivors were exposed to early in their lives. *Identity socializations* influenced survivor's *identity exploration and formation,* and opportunities for congruence later contributed to the healing strategies within the **trauma response**. The high waves of the water represent the **power and**

privileges held by the aggressor as the sexual violence event transpired. It is also possible that aggressors continued to hold higher **power and privilege** following the sexual encounter since most of these attributes were assigned to the aggressors because of their race, gender, and physical strength. Survivors, on the other hand, may have been subjected to continuous *emotional burden* due to their encounters with the systems of oppression as a result of their underrepresented identities. For sexual trauma survivors at the stage of trauma integration, the sexual violence incident was associated with increased self-awareness and intentional engagement in positive self-talk so as to maintain a positive self-worth and body awareness, and image.

The rough water and its high waves may have continued to exist as survivors engaged in the healing journey from sexual trauma and continued to navigate the roles of **power and privilege** within their **sociocultural contexts and socializations**. As survivors weathered the storm, sometimes the water was smooth and helped them to savor the **moments of relief**; at other times it may have caused a temporary imbalance in response to larger waves associated with the greater **power and privileges** of those around them, leading survivors to experience an *emotional burden*.

In general, the healing journey from sexual trauma is best understood by intentional efforts and processes that allowed participants to see beyond the trauma experience and use the traumatic experience to *authentically* represent their identities and their values. Figure 6 below is a visual representation of the boat, its structures, the water and the cloud representing the healing journey from sexual trauma.

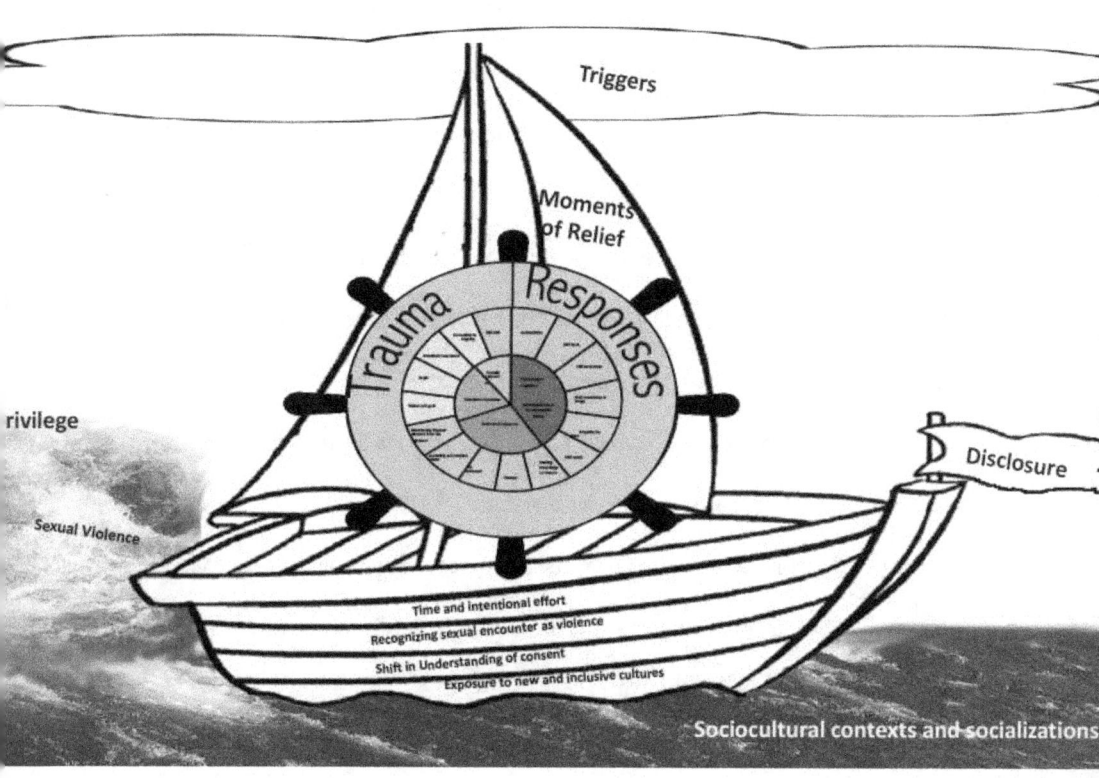

Shift in Understanding of Consent

After a sexual encounter incident, survivors began to sense that this sexual encounter was not voluntary, and that they were not in full agreement about engaging in the sexual act. However, the non-inclusive definition of consent learned from their **sociocultural contexts and socializations**, initially informed how they started to question their experience and their perception of how the sexual encounter happened. In particular, male-identifying survivors questioned their experience and attempted to interpret their sexual encounter as desirability instead of violence. The limited education around consent and sexual violence within queer relationships also contributed to the confusion around naming survivors' sexual encounter with their aggressor as violence and as traumatic. Until survivors started making a shift in their understanding of consent, they may have interpreted their actions during the sexual violence encounter as complicit, therefore believing they must have agreed to it or wanted it. This self-doubt and self-blame and questioning of their experience continued until survivors made an attempt to explore more about the sexual encounter and the meaning of consent. This exploration included **disclosure** of the sexual encounter to those significant to them, including consulting professionals and service providers. Moreover, the major uprising of social justice movements such as the #MeToo Movement helped clarify the distinction between saying "Yes!" and not saying "No!" to a sexual encounter.

Disclosures that resulted in validation and normalization were perceived as *social support* survivors received from their significant others and/or professionals. These experiences of naming the sexual encounter as violence and normalizing trauma helped survivors shift their understanding of consent. This shift in understanding of consent involved questioning the learned definition of what it means to be sexually violated, who gets sexually victimized, and what and who takes the responsibility when sexual violence occurs. In this process, survivors were able to positively transform their understanding of consent and start naming their experience as traumatic. The shift in understanding of consent led to the recognition of the sexual encounter as nonconsensual and as violence that happened to them instead of as an act that they wanted, were complicit in, and/or something they felt was desirable.

Recognizing Sexual Encounter as Violence

Once participants were able to transform their views of consent, they were able to name the sexual violence incident as violent and traumatic. This recognition of the sexual encounter as violence helped survivors to name what happened to them and focus on their **trauma responses** with intentionality. The process of recognizing the sexual encounter as violence involved the survivors' effort to accept and normalize their experience as trauma and was best supported when survivors were able to get support from others. At times, once survivors shifted their understanding of consent, they may have consulted with their *social support* system so they could validate and confirm their new understanding of the traumatic experience.

When the outcome of these disclosures became *victim questioning,* it led to feeling unheard, unseen, and unvalued. This feeling of not being valued intersected with the survivors' encounter with the system and may have contributed to survivors' *emotional burden* as they attempted to advocate for themselves and educate others about sexual violence and its prevalence across different identities. This then led survivors to spend time and effort navigating the negative *somatic responses* and *emotional responses* of trauma rather than focusing on healing strategies. Survivors surrounded by individuals who were able to help them name and normalize their experience as sexual trauma were able to engage in *behavioral* and *psychological responses* so they could begin their healing journey.

Time and Intentional Effort

After recognizing the sexual encounter as violence, survivors were able to recognize the emotional and somatic responses and intentionally invest effort and energy into focusing on helpful strategies. This intentional effort allowed survivors to identify healing strategies applicable to them so they could keep hoisting and adjusting the sail to continue their journey and maintain an even keel. As a result, intentional effort and emphasis on helping strategies assisted them by transforming their self-beliefs and understanding of trauma.

The simple passage of time itself did not necessarily contribute to healing from sexual trauma. Over time, however, survivors were able to make intentional decisions to prioritize and allocate their time to processing sexual trauma as they continued to give meaning to it. The passage of time was also helpful in creating opportunities and exposure to new information about trauma, such as the normalization of sexual violence and a new definition of consensual sex following the #MeToo Movement, which helped them externalize their traumatic experience. These social justice movements were also important as survivors explored and formed their intersecting identities, and this in turn helped survivors to be *authentic*. As time passed, survivors' intentional effort helped them to focus on helpful *behavioral responses* and recognize the self-damaging *psychological responses* to trauma so they could work on making a positive shift.

Exposure to New and Inclusive Cultures

One of the significant positive shifts for survivors of sexual trauma from underrepresented groups was *authenticity*. Survivors' *authenticity* was facilitated by their active effort to continue to explore the **power and privilege** they held as they interacted with their **sociocultural contexts and socialization** factors. This exposure to new and inclusive cultures created opportunities for survivors to question existing non-inclusive and discriminating norms reinforced by their *family culture and upbringing* as well as the *identity socializations* associated with their underrepresented identities. The exposure to new and inclusive cultures could have been a result of survivors' efforts to change their location and move out of their place of origin and/or change their social group to help them develop a new sense of community with more *social support*. Through survivors' efforts to question these existing norms, they were able to explore and form their identities congruent with who they felt they were and the values they held. This congruence in turn led to a positive trauma response by promoting a full acceptance of self and integration of trauma into their *authentic self*.

Trauma Response

Sexual violence survivors' **trauma responses** happened following and/or alongside their process of shifting their understanding of consent and recognizing their sexual encounter as violence. The <u>immediate to ongoing</u> *somatic responses* and the *shame and guilt* of the *emotional responses* were often the initial trauma reactions that informed survivors that the sexual act was not consensual. As a result, these *somatic responses* and *emotional responses* to sexual trauma may have occurred as participants transformed their understanding of consent and recognized their sexual encounter as violent and traumatic. These negative trauma reactions were also related to self-blame and self-doubt as survivors questioned their experience and perception during the sexual violence encounter. Figure 7 below illustrates the cycle of **trauma response** and survivors' act of steering the wheel of negative responses to trauma towards the positive and healing ones.

Figure 7

The Cycle of Sexual Trauma Response

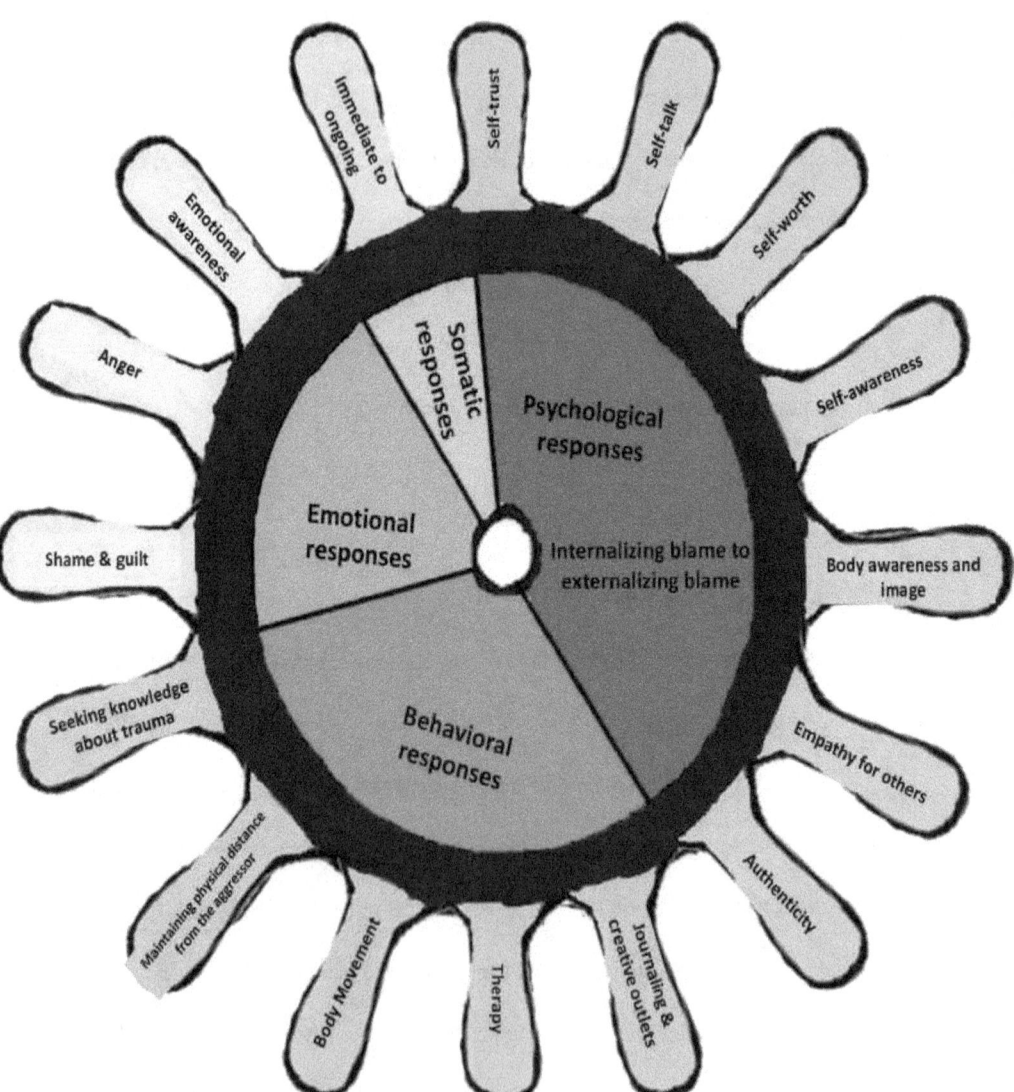

The Wheel of Trauma Response

I used the boat's wheel to represent the cycle of **trauma response**. The wheel shows the survivors' effort to ensure that the healing strategies continue to hold more weight and presence in their journey of healing than the negative **trauma responses**. The act of shifting and balancing **trauma responses** represented participants' effort to steer the boat towards a smoother water and maintain the sail hoist through the experiences of **moments of relief**.

The **trauma response** is a cycle that circulates like a wheel and involves ongoing *somatic responses, emotional responses, psychological responses,* and *behavioral responses.* This **trauma response** cycle involves several positive shifts survivors made in their thinking and feeling and added behavioral skills to help them heal from sexual trauma. Survivors' trauma response began with visible and invisible *somatic responses* during and after the encounter with sexual violence. Visible *somatic responses* like panic attacks could occur on an ongoing basis as survivors encountered triggers such as sexual intimacy attempts in new relationships and/or their aggressor's attempt to contact them without their consent.

The *somatic responses* during the violence, mostly the "freeze" trauma response, led participants to question and doubt their experience and delay the process of naming the experience as traumatic because they perceived this "freeze" as being complicit and agreeing to the sexual act. Until survivors were able to acquire knowledge on general trauma responses of fight, flight and freeze, the confusion around their perceived responsibility prior and during the sexual encounter continued, leading to an *emotional response* of *shame and guilt.* Through intentional effort and *seeking knowledge on trauma*, survivors could transform the *emotional response* of *shame and guilt* and anger (that later transformed into righteous anger) into a *psychological response* of self-trust. Trusting their memory and perception leading up to, during, and shortly after the sexual violence encounter helped survivors start externalizing and assigning blame to the aggressor. The significant process in the transformation of self-blame and self-doubt to positive self-worth and self-talk was also facilitated by the process of shifting from internalizing self-blame to externalizing the blame.

The process of INTERNALIZING BLAME TO EXTERNALIZING BLAME helped survivors trust themselves as they continued to develop their positive self-awareness and self-worth and contributed to the experience of internal moments of relief. The *behavioral responses* signify survivors' engagement in intentional healing skills such as *body movements, therapy, seeking knowledge about trauma,* and use of *journaling and creative outlets* to express themselves as well as to externalize blame regarding the sexual trauma. As depicted in Figure 7, the cycle of **trauma response** involves a continuous act of balancing the negative **trauma responses** with positive **trauma responses** so that the healing responses to trauma outweighed the negative ones.

As survivors keep steering the wheel of the boat, they focus on their knowledge of healing **trauma responses** that helped them maintain the balance and direction of their boat and hoist the sail. They also remained emotionally aware, so they know and feel when their boat is off balance and/or heading in a direction that leads to an imbalance. This steering and balancing required survivors to make shifts towards healing **trauma responses** when encountering negative **trauma responses**. Below is a description of these shifts that contribute to healing from sexual trauma.

Somatic responses. Part of the negative **trauma response** cycle involved the experience of *somatic responses*. The magnitude of these *somatic responses* ranged from a moment of "freeze" during the sexual violence encounter to full panic attack symptoms that were experienced as the sexual violence was occurring and reappeared when survivors were triggered. These triggers could have been related to the aggressor's attempt to contact the survivor and the threat of perceived inability to maintain physical distance from the aggressor following the sexual violence. Other triggers may have involved initial sexual intimacy encounters as survivors attempted to establish new intimate sexual relationships. These triggers led to the ongoing *somatic responses* leading survivors to feel shame about their inability to control them. When *somatic responses* held greater weight, the spike of the wheel representing the negative *trauma responses* became salient creating an imbalance of the boat and leading survivors to exert more energy to focus on healing strategies to regain their balance.

Emotional responses. Survivors' *emotional responses* to sexual violence included *shame and guilt* and anger. *Shame and guilt* were felt when self-doubt and self-blame were heightened surrounding the survivors' perceived role and responsibility during the sexual encounter. Shame could be felt for perceived complicity and guilt could be felt for not fighting back, not saying no, or engaging in a sexual encounter with someone survivors would not approve of if they were given a choice. Shame could also be associated with the perceived inability to control the ongoing *somatic symptoms* that were experienced in the presence of others.

Anger, on the other hand, was a two-fold. On the one hand, participants felt anger towards their aggressor and the system that gave the aggressor more **power and privilege**. As survivors started to name and recognize their trauma, however, anger shifted to a righteous anger that was more empowering and assisted them to assert themselves, so survivors started to set and maintain their boundaries in romantic and other intimate relationships. Survivors' ability to develop their *emotional awareness* assisted them in recognizing the need for intentional efforts to shift towards healing strategies; these may have included holding on to empowering righteous anger, and externalizing blame instead of continuing to feel ashamed and guilty about their perceived role during the sexual violence encounter.

Behavioral responses. Once survivors of sexual trauma were able to recognize their *somatic* and *emotional responses*, they could engage in the act of "doing" that was helpful in transforming negative **trauma responses** to more positive ones. These *behavioral responses* included *maintaining physical distance from their aggressor*. Without maintaining physical distance from the aggressor, survivors may have feared for their safety. The threat to their safety could have been exacerbated by any trigger that heightened their perceived inability to have the choice to maintain their physical distance from the aggressor. This trigger included fear of another physical encounter with their aggressor because they shared a communal space and/or used similar social media platforms that narrowed the perceived physical distance and safety from the aggressor.

As a means of externalizing blame, survivors engaged in *journaling and creative outlets*. This included writing nonfiction, song notes and lyrics, poetry, and keeping a personal journal to reflect on their experience of healing from sexual trauma. These *journaling and creative outlets* were also helpful for recognizing, releasing, and externalizing *shame and guilt* and anger associated with their traumatic experience. Another intentional action that survivors of sexual trauma used was seeking ways to educate themselves about trauma and trauma responses. This journey of *seeking knowledge about trauma* helped survivors to recognize the trauma reactions of fight, flight and freeze. This knowledge helped them shift their feeling of shame for not saying no or not fighting back to having an awareness of how their body responded to trauma. Specifically for male-identifying sexual trauma survivors who were at the early stages of their identity exploration and formation at the time of their encounter with sexual violence, the act of *seeking knowledge about trauma* was helpful to build empathy towards others who may have experienced trauma. Seeking and obtaining knowledge about trauma was also important as sexual trauma survivors in underrepresented groups developed their understanding of systemic oppression.

Body movement, one of the *behavioral responses,* including yoga, hiking, camping, etc., also helped survivors to develop a positive body awareness and image as well as self-worth and *authenticity.* Survivors may have found one or all of these *body movements* helpful to experience **internal relief** from the sexual trauma. *Body movement* created an opportunity to focus within the survivors' body that encountered the sexual violence and engage in creating a positive body awareness and image and building self-awareness. Engagement in *therapy* may also have been helpful to survivors as it facilitated their self-awareness, self-worth, *emotional awareness,* and encouraged them to focus on *behavioral responses* that contributed to healing from sexual trauma.

Psychological responses. The *psychological responses* to trauma were mostly characterized by the positive shift survivors made as they healed from sexual trauma. Shortly after recognizing the sexual encounter as violence and during the active stages of *somatic responses* and *emotional responses,* survivors experienced self-doubt, self-blame, and negative self-image. However, as participants engaged in helpful *behavioral responses,* they started to shift the INTERNALIZED BLAME TO EXTERNALIZED BLAME so that blame was shifted towards both their aggressor and the enabling system. The externalizing of blame was beneficial in two ways. First, survivors were able to rightfully assign blame to their aggressor without justifying the actions of the aggressor and blaming themselves for perceived complicity during the sexual violence encounter. Second, they were able to recognize the system and norms that enabled their aggressor by normalizing the oppression of those who hold less **power and privilege**. In this case, survivors were able to recognize the existing **sociocultural systems and socializations** and shift their actions from conforming to advocating. The change from conforming to advocating assisted sexual trauma survivors in underrepresented groups to question existing systems of "isms," develop their awareness of social justice issues, and engage in advocacy in an attempt to create an accepting and inclusive social environment that allowed them and others with underrepresented identities to be *authentic*.

Authenticity helped survivors of sexual trauma to experience **moments of relief**. The experience of *authenticity* came with survivors' ability to fully and freely engage in *identity exploration and formation* as well as safety and relief related to the exposure to cultures that are inclusive and accepting of individuals in underrepresented groups. The barriers to *authenticity* may have included fear of uncontrolled *somatic responses* when triggered and general fear for safety especially when holding intersections of underrepresented identities in a sociocultural context that was not accepting and inclusive.

Among the *psychological responses* to sexual trauma was also the survivor's intentional decision to make a positive shift towards their body awareness and image. Lack of and/or minimal body awareness and negative body image contributed to *shame and guilt* following sexual trauma. To heal from sexual trauma, survivors needed to have a positive image towards their body and recognize their body as resilient and deserving to be honored and loved.

Similarly, continuous efforts of increasing self-awareness were associated with healing. Self-awareness enabled survivors to recognize the source of each of their **trauma responses** and helped them to intentionally focus on the healing strategies. Moreover, as survivors developed their self-awareness, their intentionality around *authentically* presenting themselves increased.

One of the significant shifts in the *psychological responses* that contributed to the healing journey was self-trust. Often, especially for survivors who were questioning their perception during the sexual violence and were unable to name and accept the sexual encounter as traumatic, the shift from self-doubt to self-trust was essential. The shift towards trusting oneself helped survivors to assure themselves even as others were questioning the traumatic nature of the sexual encounter with their aggressor. This in turn helped them to rely on their perceptions of the sexual violence, to name, normalize and validate their experience instead of questioning it.

Positive self-worth was also a prominent factor in the healing journey from sexual trauma. There is a possibility that sexual trauma survivors in this study, due to their underrepresented identities and the lesser **power and privilege** assigned to these identities by the survivors' sociocultural contexts, may have felt undeserving of love and therefore limited in their ability to be authentically themselves. It is also possible that survivors faced insults by their aggressor following the sexual violence encounter that targeted their race, body, gender, etc., thus adding to the negative self-worth. As a result, the shift towards a positive self-worth that came with balanced self-awareness, positive body awareness and image, and positive self-talk, played a significant role in the healing of sexual trauma survivors.

The shift from negative self-talk to positive self-talk also helped survivors to emphasize the intentional efforts they were making towards their healing. These self-recognized positive shifts towards self-affirming self-talk allowed survivors to recognize and acknowledge the progress they had made towards healing. A positive shift towards self-affirming self-talk also provided an opportunity to increase the balanced and positive self-awareness, body awareness and image, and self-worth that made healing from sexual trauma possible.

Moreover, as survivors engaged in the *behavioral response* of *seeking knowledge about trauma*, they made a self-recognized positive shift towards a deeper understanding of the pain associated with sexual violence. This deeper connection with other survivors of trauma contributed to the survivors' empathy for others who were victims of sexual violence. This shift in empathy for others was a conscious recognition of an emotional connection with other survivors of sexual violence.

In sum, the cycle of **trauma response** represented by the boat's wheel consists of the intentional shifts in emotions, thoughts, and skills as survivors of sexual trauma attempted to heal from sexual trauma. This attempt of healing happened while survivors anticipated sporadic encounters with triggers that elicited negative somatic and emotional responses. These triggers and the encounters with higher waves of **power and privilege** held by others require survivors to hold on to the helping handles of the wheel during turbulences so they can continue to maintain a float. This leads survivors to keep their hands on the wheel as they steer their healing boat towards a smoother water. Within this **trauma response** cycle, survivors were also tasked with assessing and balancing the negative trauma responses with positive ones. **Moments of relief** occurred when survivors were able to emphasize, attain, and maintain healing *behavioral responses* and *psychological responses* that outweighed the negative *somatic* and *emotional responses* to sexual trauma.

Disclosure

The act of disclosing an unwanted sexual encounter, represented as the flag attached to the boat, involved two major components: the *intrapersonal considerations of disclosure* and the *interpersonal outcomes of disclosure*. The survivors' *purpose of disclosure* of the sexual violence encounter ranged from wishing to gain support from others to a desire to advocate by being a voice for other sexual trauma survivors. Survivors also disclosed their sexual trauma for the purpose of educating those who may otherwise have the potential to be victimized and/or those who question victims of sexual violence. At times, initial disclosure of the experience of sexual trauma may have been unintentionally expressed through noticeable and uncontrolled *emotional responses* like anger and/or *somatic responses* such as panic attacks. This anger and panic attach could result in unintentional disclosure of sexual trauma leading survivors to personally consider the *purpose of disclosure* so they could shift from unintentional disclosure to intentional disclosure. Intentional disclosure involved the choice the survivor made to seek help from others and/or engage in advocacy so they could be a voice for others.

Once disclosure was made, the *interpersonal outcomes of disclosure* guided the **trauma response** as well as the **moments of relief**. One possible *interpersonal outcome of disclosure* was *social support*. This *social support* was obtained from romantic partners, other family members, close friends, therapists, and work colleagues who were able to help the survivor shift their understanding of consent, name the sexual encounter as violence and traumatic, and validate the survivors' experience of **trauma response**. *Social support* was, therefore, related to moments of internal peace for participants that strengthened the survivors' sense of belongingness.

Another possible *interpersonal outcome of disclosure* was *victim questioning*. When questioned, survivors of sexual trauma often felt unheard, unseen, and unvalued which then led to negative emotional **trauma responses**. Although it was unpleasant, survivors who were well grounded in their knowledge of trauma and those who were able to make a positive shift in their understanding of consent and **trauma responses** could engage in discussions with those who were questioning them. These discussions around the definition of consent enabled them to come to a common understanding and allowed survivors to maintain social relations with those who questioned them instead of shutting down. However, seeking physical and relational distance from those who questioned their trauma experience was common when the preexisting relationship was not strong.

Moments of relief

Represented by the sail of the boat, the **moments of relief** served as a sign and evidence that survivors were experiencing moments of healing. These **moments of relief** were characterized by the internal peace and a feeling of lesser weight of the pain caused by the sexual trauma. **Moments of relief** could also represent the sense of freedom felt when finding relatable experiences with others who shared similar underrepresented group(s) identities and intersections of those identities.

The moments of *internal relief* were mostly related to healing moments from sexual trauma. *Internal relief* informed survivors that their intentional efforts to heal were paying off. On the other hand, *external relief* was a sense of freedom from systemic oppression. This *external relief* was experienced by survivors of sexual trauma as a result of *interpersonal and relational relief* through feeling not only heard but also understood by those around them. Moreover, *external relief* was experienced through the *societal relief* that came with observing and encountering systemic changes towards inclusivity of those in underrepresented groups. The combination of *internal and external moments of relief* instilled hope and continued to hoist the sail as the boat remained afloat and continued on this healing journey.

Summary

This chapter presented the grounded theory of healing from sexual trauma for survivors identifying as members of underrepresented groups based on their gender, race, sexual, and/or disability identity. This journey of healing is represented as a boat that keeps floating through and in spite of a storm. The water depicts the **sociocultural context and socializations** that informed and assigned a greater **power and privilege** to the aggressors at the time of the sexual violence. Hence, at the time of the sexual violence, aka the storm, participants held less **power and privilege** compared to their aggressor despite the fact that their aggressor might have held an *intersection of privileged and nonprivileged identities*.

Intentional engagement in healing strategies and helpful **trauma responses** occurred when survivors were able to make a shift in their understanding of consent and recognize the sexual encounter as an act of violence. Through this shift and recognition, often intertwined with the processes of time and intentional effort and exposure to new and inclusive cultures, sexual trauma survivors focused on helpful strategies to heal from the sexual trauma. *Social support* played a significant role in strengthening the planks of the boat and provided an opportunity for survivors to keep steering the boat's wheel towards healing **trauma responses** and outweigh the negative reactions towards trauma. These efforts led to **moments** of relief associated with healing from trauma. *Societal relief* and *interpersonal and relational relief* that provided relatable experiences led to a sense of freedom from systemic oppression. These moments of freedom, represented as *external relief,* combined with the survivors' journey of *identity exploration and formation* helped survivors to realize moments of *authenticity*.

CHAPTER 6: TRUSTWORTHINESS, LIMITATIONS, AND IMPLICATIONS

In this chapter, I will discuss the methods I used to establish data trustworthiness and will highlight the limitations that emerged in this study. I will also explain my process of reaching data saturation. Finally, I will share the implications of this study and directions for future research to build upon the grounded theory illustrated in Chapter Five. Before describing the methods of trustworthiness, limitations, and implications, however, it important to provide a brief discussion of the existing conceptual framework based on the literature reviewed in Chapter One in relation to the theory illustrated in Chapter Five.

Some studies (e.g., Enright & Rique, 2004; Prieto-Ursúa, 2021; Tracy, 1999) have indicated that forgiveness was found to be beneficial for healing from sexual trauma. In the grounded theory of the current study, however, only one participant (Tim Samson) named forgiveness as having a positive contribution to his healing journey. Tim Samson described his process of forgiving as *"This is where I feel a lot of grace and a lot of forgiveness, because a lot of these guys [aggressors] like didn't hold much power in the world, because they were very, obviously, the gay men. For the most part, we might say very obviously, feminine men."* Tim Samson's process indicated the positive role of survivor's recognition of the *intersection of privileged and underrepresented identities of the aggressor* that facilitated healing from sexual trauma. However, based on the data that emerged in this grounded theory study, Tim Samson's experience of forgiving his aggressors was singular, and insufficient to allow one to conclude the importance of forgiveness of aggressors in healing from sexual trauma. However, participants shared how shifting from internalizing blame to externalizing blame promoted self-trust, recognition of self-worth, and a shift to positive self-talk. Although this shift in blame can be interpreted as a process of survivors' self-forgiveness (Pierro et al., 2018), participants have not named this process as self-forgiveness. I therefore chose to follow the words and language used by participants to describe this process as a shift in blame rather than naming it as "self-forgiveness."

Other studies have named justice as a significant factor in healing from sexual violence (Campbell et al., 2009; Ringland, 2017; Saint & Sinko, 2019; Swanson & Szymanski, 2020). However, none of the six participants in this study reported their sexual violence encounter to the justice system. Nichole, River, and Nathan specifically talked about the *emotional burden* they experienced because of their encounter with the system, a burden that contributed to their decision not to report their experience to the police. Nichole, who identifies as a person of color, had witnessed other sexual trauma survivors experience an unpleasant outcome of reporting sexual violence to the legal system. Nichole was also explicit about their fear of encountering systemic oppression through the legal system considering the power and privilege their aggressor held as a white male with social power. River, who identifies as a white nonbinary and pansexual, had witnessed and experienced sexual violence in the hands of the police. Nathan, who identifies as a mixed-race Asian America man, explicitly stated the stereotype and systemic discrimination against "ethnic" men and his fear of being victim blamed or even considered as the aggressor because of his gender and race. For these reasons, all these three participants were adamant about not reporting their sexual violence to the legal system. These voices indicated that sexual trauma survivors in underrepresented groups encounter the justice system differently and become the direct or indirect victims of the systemic oppression that alters their decision to report sexual violence when it happens to them. As a result, for the participants of this study, the **trauma response and moments of relief** were independent of seeking and receiving perceived justice.

According to the study by Swanson and Szymanski (2020), advocacy was an important factor in empowering survivors of sexual trauma and one that contributed to healing. In this study, however, the shift from conforming to advocacy was interpreted as an *emotional burden* participants experienced as they navigated their encounter with the system. Advocacy was also related to participants' experience of questioning, educating themselves, and attempting to be a voice for themselves and others who may otherwise not have the voice to represent themselves. The dimension of conforming to advocacy was related to negative emotional experiences for participants as they navigated their sociocultural and contextual systems that can sometimes became triggers during the healing journey.

Pre-trauma resiliency skills were also cited in the literature as facilitating healing from sexual trauma (e.g., Campbell et al., 2009; Durà-Vilà et al., 2013; Newsom & Myers-Bowman, 2017; Saint & Sinko, 2019; Swanson & Szymanski, 2020). In this grounded theory, only pre-trauma sense of self was found to be significant in participants' positive shift towards UNDERSTANDING OF CONSENT and avoiding self-blame by recognizing **trauma response** and the **power and privilege** held by their aggressor. In this study, *sense of self* i.e., the understanding of identities, values, and awareness of themselves as they interacted with the rest of the world prior to the sexual violence experience, was discussed by participants as part of their *pre-trauma self and relationships.* This *sense of self* included survivors' positive shift in their understanding of consent prior to the trauma experience, and helped them to seek support from others; after naming their sexual encounter with the aggressor as violence, they were better able to focus on healing strategies.

Social connection, another significant factor in processing trauma (e.g., Durà-Vilà et al., 2013; Ringland, 2017; Sinko et al., 2021), emerged in this grounded theory study as *social support* within the *subcategory* of *interpersonal outcomes of disclosure* as well as the *relationship with others* within the *pre-trauma self*. Social connection is evident in the pre-trauma *relationship with others* that was instrumental in facilitating **disclosure of** sexual trauma and receiving *social support*.

Studies by Freedman and Enright (1996, 2017), Saint and Sinko (2019) and Campbell, et al. (2009) identified preexisting close and familial relationship with the perpetrator as a factor that negatively impacts the journey following sexual trauma. These studies indicated that incest, child abuse, and date rape resulted in increasingly negative responses to trauma. This factor was not directly related and significant to the experience of participants in this study since survivors of childhood sexual trauma were excluded from this study.

Prior studies also indicated that socioeconomic and cultural considerations were important factors for understanding the healing journey from sexual trauma (Campbell et al., 2009; Ginwright, 2018; Gomez & Gobin, 2020). When I proposed this study, I had indicated Gomez (2012)'s Cultural Betrayal Trauma Theory (CBTT) as a conceptual framework to illustrate the role of intracultural trust and pressure in underrepresented groups. In this case, survivors' efforts to report and seek justice and/or advocacy can be considered as a betrayal of this intracultural trust leading to the cultural pressures survivors experience. CBTT asserts that the shared understanding and camaraderie within members of underrepresented groups makes it difficult for survivors to disclose their sexual trauma and seek justice when the aggressor is within the same underrepresented group. In this grounded theory, however, only one participant (Christina) shared that two of the sexual violence encounters were with aggressors within her same sexual orientation group. All the other participants shared that their aggressors held **power and privilege** because of their race, gender, physical strength and/or social and positional power. As a result, there was not enough data in this study to support CBTT and explain the journey of healing sexual trauma through this theory. This study did, however, highlight the impact of **power and privilege**, shaped by the **sociocultural contexts and socialization**, on **trauma responses** and experiences of **moments of relief** for sexual trauma survivors in underrepresented groups.

Below are descriptions of the methods for establishing trustworthiness, the limitations of the current study, implications of the findings, and directions for future research.

Establishing Trustworthiness

Lincoln and Guba (2007) suggested four pillars of establishing trustworthiness in a qualitative inquiry: credibility for internal validity, transferability for external validity, dependability for reliability, and confirmability for objectivity (pp. 18-19). To establish credibility, I used member checking, prolonged engagement, triangulation, and peer debriefing. To establish transferability, I generated thick and rich descriptive data and used reflexivity. To establish dependability, I used inquiry auditing. To establish confirmability, I used inquiry auditing and member checking. Collectively, these methods of establishing trustworthiness address all four "parallel criteria of trustworthiness" identified by Lincoln and Guba (2007, p. 18).

Member checking

I used member checking as a method to establish credibility and transferability of the data co-constructed with participants and to formulate this grounded theory of healing from sexual trauma. After formulating the grounded theory described in Chapter Five, I sent an email (see Appendix M) to each of the six participants with an attachment of a file titled "conceptual maps and summary of the theory" (see Appendix N). In the attachment, I included the two images in Chapter Five that were created to illustrate the theory of "weathering the storm: the journey of healing from sexual trauma." I also included a brief summary of the theory that described the major themes within these images. In the email, I offered my availability for a discussion and/or to answer any questions participants may have as they respond to the member checking questions.

During the member checking I asked participants five questions:

1. Is there anything about these images and the descriptions that resonates with you?
2. Is there anything I got wrong?
3. Is there anything that needs to be added?
4. Is there anything that needs to be changed or removed?
5. What are your overall impressions?

Moreover, since I had been using text messages as a primary means of contact with four participants, I followed up my member checking email with a text to inform them about the email and reiterate my availability to answer any questions they may have as they read the summary of the theory and answered the five above questions.

Member checking results. So far, I have received feedback from Tim Samson, Christina, Nathan and River for the member check questions. In his response to the member checking questions, Tim Samson stated that "The narrative account matches my experience very well." Christina also stated that "I feel that your description is an accurate representation of the information received during the interviews. I would not change or remove any part." She further elaborated her thoughts on the theory by stating "I really liked how you put the points of healing on the steering wheel of the boat. I feel that this is very representative of how healing is, in the cyclical form combined with moving the boat to calmer seas." River shared a summary of her thoughts on what resonate with her as "I like the images with the wave and the wheel, I think it makes sense. I find it important that everyone's journey is different, and everyone's healing is different. And this is a good representation of showing that."

In answering the question of what could be added, Christina shared that "I think the only thing I would have added is that healing from this trauma is partially a choice. You have to let go of anger to heal, whether that is anger towards the assault or towards the system. This can be difficult, and it can be seen as part of the process for healing." Tim Samson also shared "The images are helpful, but I *personally* resonated more with the textual account of the data. The font in the wheel was hard for me to read."

When sharing their overall impression, Christina shared "My overall impressions are that this is a great, accurate representation of what someone may have gone through with their healing process. I think that the metaphor of the boat in the sea is a good one. You did well explaining the different parts of the image and how they are representative of the healing process for someone with intersecting identities." Similarly, Tim Samson added "Overall, it is validating to see my individual experience qualitatively represented in a set of group-collected data!" Nathan did not answer each member checking question but provided his overall impression on the theory as "I looked over what you have, and I think they are great! The triggers, moments of relief, and responses with the sailboat really spoke to me. I like that triggers were in the shape of a cloud, because it often does feel that way. Like a storm roll in and blows my life in a direction where I have to steer into trauma responses."

Prolonged engagement

Another method I used to account for credibility was prolonged engagement. Once participants reached out expressing their willingness and interest to participate in this study, I communicated with them, both via email and text (based on their preferred means of communication) to gather background information and determine their eligibility, schedule both rounds of interviews, collect artwork to represent their journey with sexual trauma, and for member checking. The minimum time I spent with a participant, when combining the time spent during the two rounds of interviews, ranged from 83 minutes to 132 minutes.

During both rounds of interviews, I explained the purpose of my research, procedures of managing and making decisions, unforeseeable risks and crisis during the interview, and invited them to ask any questions they may have throughout their engagement with this study. I answered any questions that arose during these interviews including procedures of interviews and member checking as well as reasons for my focus on sexual trauma in underrepresented groups. I listened actively and reflected what I was hearing from them to confirm and elaborate their description of their experiences and process of surviving sexual trauma. Participants shared their gratitude for the opportunity to share their experience of sexual trauma by reiterating their belief in the need to keep talking about both the prevalence and impact of sexual trauma in underrepresented groups. Nathan shared his commitment to participate in this study as a way to advocate for and give voice to male sexual trauma survivors. River disclosed that one of the moments of relief for her was during the first-round interview since it was a moment she was able to clearly articulate her journey with sexual trauma without the surfacing of negative somatic and emotional responses. Tim Samson also reflected on his participation as "it was my pleasure and privilege 😊"

Triangulation

I also used triangulation to establish credibility of the data generated for this grounded theory study. I asked participants to share an artwork/artifact that represented their journey of surviving sexual trauma. All of the six participants submitted at least one art that represent their journey of healing from sexual trauma. These arts included poems, essay, photo, and song lyrics. These artwork/artifact pieces submitted by participants were included in part and/or in full to supplement the themes that emerged during the first and second rounds of analyses. The full versions of artwork/artifacts can be found under Appendix J.

Peer debriefing

I did not initially plan to use peer debriefing as a method of establishing trustworthiness. However, I had the opportunity to discuss the emerging categories and subcategories as well as the initial and final conceptual maps with peers who are in the Counselor Education and Supervision doctoral program here at the University of Montana. I was also able to share these emerging data with professionals outside of the counseling profession. Lincoln and Guba (2007) stated that peer debriefing is "exposing oneself to a disinterested professional peer to 'keep the inquirer honest,' assist in developing working hypotheses, develop and test the emerging design, and obtain emotional catharsis" (p. 19). To this end, I presented my dissertation proposal to the COUN 685 internship class, a class of ten doctoral students in Counselor Education and Supervision and a faculty supervisor. During these discussions, I was able to receive feedback from my peers about data representation in the initial conceptual maps, debrief on the challenges of achieving maximum variation, and discuss emerging themes.

I also held a one-to-one consultation meeting with a doctoral student peer who was conducting a grounded theory study on a different topic, and we discussed my own process of engaging with the data. In addition, I used two of my writing session appointments with the University of Montana Writing Center to share the categories that emerged and initial conceptual maps. These meetings were helpful to me to reflect my process out loud as I created connections within, between and among categories I identified. These peer debriefings were helpful for emotional catharsis and for reflecting on the developing hypothesis for this grounded theory.

Inquiry auditing

To establish dependability and confirmability, I used inquiry auditing. Dr. Veronica Johnson, my dissertation chair, served as my inquiry auditor for this study. Dr. Johnson and I met weekly for at least an hour from Fall 2021 to Summer 2023 to discuss this dissertation study. During these five semesters, Dr. Johnson provided mentorship and reviewed drafts and completed sections of this study at each stage of its progress. She reviewed each theme that emerged during both rounds of analysis and discussed the process of identifying categories, subcategories, properties, and dimensions. In addition, we collaborated on several initial conceptual maps following the first- and second rounds of analyses. Dr. Johnson's mentorship, consultation, and advice was critical throughout the development and conclusion of this study.

I also consulted with Dr. Kirsten Murray, one of the dissertation committee members, on sound qualitative inquiry for developing this grounded theory as well as the formulation of initial categories and subcategories, properties and dimensions that were emerging during both the first-round and second-round analyses. Dr. Murray's support and mentorship were instrumental in helping me identify major emerging themes, identify gaps and develop interview questions for both rounds of interviews.

Generating thick and rich descriptions

To establish transferability, I generated thick and rich descriptions of the data that emerged during the two rounds of analyses. To this end, in addition to providing clear and explanatory definitions for each **category**, *subcategory*, *property*, <u>dimension</u> and PROCESS, I added direct quotes to represent participants' voices that support these themes. I also included artwork/artifacts that supported these direct quotes and the emerging themes. These thick and rich descriptions allowed this grounded theory to come to life so that readers could understand and then evaluate the transferability of the data themselves.

Reflexivity

I used reflexivity to establish the transferability of the data co-constructed with the participants in this study. As a researcher who identifies as a black woman, I was cognizant of the role my visible identity could play in the way participants discussed their experience and process. For instance, Nichole's statement of "It feels almost too obvious [power the aggressor has due to race and gender identity] to say. Yeah. It was so weird" could be related to a shared BIPOC identity I had with the participant. Moreover, Nathan's hesitance in describing women's power and privilege such as "and please forgive me if that's ignorant because I could be completely wrong" and/or "at least in my experience I'm not gonna generalize [to] anyone because I think it's wrong to generalize" could be associated with the power and privilege I held in the room as someone who identifies as a woman. To address these hesitance and assumptions of shared experiences, I asked follow up clarifying questions. For instance, I asked Nichole about what seemed obvious in their experience with white men. For Nathan, I thanked him for sharing his perspective and experience, and provided assurance that his voice is important. In addition, during the after interview debrief, Sophie shared her disagreement with the use of the word "healing" in relation to trauma recovery. She stated that the word healing implies to the responsibility of trauma recovery falls onto the survivor while the burden of change should have been the aggressors and the larger social system. In accordance with this feedback, I used "moments of relief" and "moments of relief and empowerment" to indicate specific instances of internal and external relief that were indicative of trauma recovery. I also used the following strategies of reflexivity throughout my study.

First, I created a memo during the interviews and used this data to note specific participants' expression such as tone of voice, silence, hesitation, and emphasis as they described their experience with sexual trauma. This memo was integrated into the corresponding quotes to bring the quotes to life and emphasize the nonverbal communications during the interviews. Second, I created a folder titled "conceptual maps" to organize and note the evolution of the initial conceptual maps that were designed to illustrate the healing journey from sexual trauma. As shown in Appendix K, during the first-round analysis, the conceptual maps evolved from a map showing complex relationships among the categories, subcategories, properties, and dimensions to a simpler and less forced presentation of the relationships among these themes. This allowed me to identify gaps in the data during the first-round analysis and to develop second-round interview questions. Similarly, several initial maps were created during the second-round analysis (see Appendix L) as I was developing a working hypothesis that represented the healing from sexual trauma. Third, I remained cognizant of my own power and positionality as I interacted with the participants. To this end, before each round of interviews, I made sure to establish and strengthen rapport, to actively listen and to use my reflection skills to confirm and clarify participants' disclosures. Fourth, as I was conducting the first and second rounds of analysis and selecting quotes, I made sure to re-review the accurate representation of the quotes under the identified themes. This required me to zoom in and out and revisit the focused codes and axial codes. My inquiry auditor was instrumental in helping me identify my biases during this process, allowing me to slow down and follow the data with clarity.

Achieving saturation

Saturation is achieved when a new data analysis does not provide additional information to the existing categories, subcategories, properties, and dimensions (Chun Tie et al., 2019). This means the "new data being collected becomes redundant and, in interviews, for example, 'the researcher begins to hear comments again and again'" (Saunders et al., 2018, p. 1896). This informs the researcher that they have reached saturation. During my first interviews with the participants, I noticed that some of the major themes I identified were becoming redundant and no new information was being added to the categories, subcategories, properties, and dimensions. For instance, information regarding disclosure and its outcomes, the role of social, cultural, and contextual factors in shaping power and privilege, and most of the components of trauma responses were discussed by participants in great detail during the first-round interview. During the second-round analysis, participants mostly confirmed those major themes, and new information was used to elaborate on and clarify these themes.

Following the first-round analysis, Dr. Johnson and I, in consultation with Dr. Murray, closely analyzed the gaps during first-round analyses and developed questions to identify processes that helped connect and establish relationships within and among the categories that had emerged. We also added inquiries based on the gaps we identified such as questions about the role of time. The data collected during the second round of interviews was instrumental in developing new processes as well as clarifying and supporting the existing categories.

By the eleventh (of 12) interview, I noticed that there was no new information added to the **categories**, *subcategories*, *properties*, and dimensions, but rather that all information confirmed and supplemented what I identified based on the previous ten interviews. I did not feel the need to add another participant for theoretical sampling because the information identified during the two rounds of interviews with six participants was becoming repetitive. As a result, in line with Charmaz's (2012) definition of theoretical sampling ["sampling for development of a theoretical category, not sampling for population representation"] (p. 2), no additional participants were needed to satisfy theoretical sampling. However, it is important to recognize the potential to identify more and new information by interviewing additional participants from other underrepresented groups outside of the identities represented in this study.

Limitations

Despite my effort to establish trustworthiness, limitations regarding maximum variation and member checking did emerge in this study. Although I was able to achieve the proposed maximum variation after interviewing six participants, others with identities situated in additional underrepresented groups could have added to the diversity of the data. For instance, regarding disability status, despite my continuous attempts to reach out to different groups representing the disability community (see Appendix G), this study does not include representation of participants with physical and/or sensory disability. This would have added to the diversity of knowledge regarding the interaction of disability status with healing from sexual trauma.

Moreover, the sample representation in my study for the Black, Indigenous, and People of Color (BIPOC) community is limited to survivors who identify as Asian, Filipino

American, and Hispanic White. Although these voices were important, and their representation was impactful, considering the diversity within the BIPOC community, additional representation of racial diversity would have added to the depth of the data I collected. In addition, on sampling, I distributed the call for participation to agencies and professionals I was familiar with and/or can access indirectly through the professionals I am familiar with. This limited potential for disseminating the call to a larger geographical area within the United States.

Moreover, after contacting each of the six participants for member check, at the time of writing the conclusion of this study, I was only able to receive feedback from Tim Samson, Christina, Nathan, and River. This partial response from participants may have impacted the transferability and credibility of the data.

Implications

This grounded theory of the journey of healing from sexual trauma helps to explain factors that assisted participants in creating meaning from their sexual violence experience. Here, I describe the implications of this grounded theory for survivors of sexual trauma, mental health service providers, educators and supervisors of mental health professionals, members of the justice system, and for friends, family and/or others in relationships with survivors of sexual trauma.

For survivors of sexual trauma

The experience of naming, accepting, and normalizing sexual trauma was identified as a significant step towards a survivors' ability to use time and exert intentional effort towards trauma responses. Openness and educating oneself about consent, both in heteronormative gender and sexual orientation identities and queer communities, is valuable for being able to recognize the sexual encounter as violence and traumatic. This normalization and developing knowledge about consent was especially fundamental for survivors in the masculine gender spectrum and those identifying as queer. The experience of naming, accepting and normalizing the encounter with sexual violence helped participants to feel validated and minimize self-doubt and blame associated with survivors' perceived responsibility before and after the sexual violence.

Also instrumental to their healing journey was survivors' shift from self-blame and *shame and guilt* to blaming and transforming to righteous anger towards their aggressor and the enabling system. Hence, this shift helped survivors to invest their time and energy on healing strategies instead of feeling stuck in negative trauma reactions. Finding a social support group that validates both the experience of sexual trauma as well as the emotional burden due to the encounter with the system was also valuable for survivors' experiences with internal and external moments of relief. As a result, sexual trauma survivors would benefit from establishing and maintaining a social support group, while also minimizing their exposure to victim questioning whenever possible.

It is also beneficial for survivors to recognize and normalize the cyclical nature of trauma response. This recognition could help them to gain insights about stuck points within the negative trauma responses such as *shame and guilt,* panic attacks, and negative self-worth, self-talk or body image. Naming and recognizing the trauma cycle would also be helpful to emphasize positive behavioral responses such as *body movement, journaling and creative outlets, therapy, seeking knowledge on trauma,* and *maintaining physical distance from the aggressor.* These behavioral responses would assist survivors in shifting to positive <u>self-talk</u> and <u>self-worth</u> and increased <u>self-awareness</u>. Survivors' genuine exploration and formation of their intersecting identities was also foundational in developing an authentic self, and was thus important for participants to experience moments of relief.

For mental health service providers

When working with survivors of sexual trauma in underrepresented groups, it is important for mental health service providers to help their clients become educated about consent. Naming and normalizing the non-inclusive nature of existing education and messaging on consent and the gap in its applicability in queer relationships can help survivors recognize trauma reactions. This, in turn, will help them develop a new understanding of consent, name the experience as traumatic, and then be able to focus on positive emotional, psychological, and behavioral responses to sexual trauma. The naming and normalizing of the prevalence of sexual violence among male-identifying individuals is also important so that male sexual trauma survivors feel heard and valued, and receive the attention they deserve.

The clear and accurate understanding of consent helps shift survivors' initial tendency of blaming and doubting themselves as well as questioning their reaction and role as the sexual violence encounter transpired. Thus, psychoeducation and mental health professionals' ability to name and normalize the sexual violence experience would be helpful for survivors to start their journey of self-trust and externalizing the blame.

Importantly, the emotional burden experienced by sexual trauma survivors in underrepresented groups due to their encounters with the system should be recognized and normalized in the counseling room. The barriers to reporting sexual violence (namely, the greater power and privilege of the aggressor and the system and norms tailored towards those with higher power and privilege) all need to be recognized during the counseling process. In the counseling room, it is important to target survivors' experience of immediate to ongoing somatic systems and *shame and guilt* as well as anger, and to help survivors strengthen their *emotional awareness*. Normalizing trauma response as a cycle that potentially revolves around both negative and positive responses, could be helpful to sexual trauma survivors.

In this grounded theory, the sociocultural contexts and socializations were found to play a significant role in the exploration and formation of intersecting identities. Combined with societal factors that influenced identity socializations, the family upbringing and culture impacted survivors' ability to be their authentic self. Authenticity, one of the positive trauma responses, was found to help survivors experience moments of relief. Moreover, the power and privilege both the aggressor and the survivor held prior to, during, and following the sexual violence determines participants' decisions about seeking justice, advocating for themselves and others, and their response to trauma. As a result, it is essential for mental health service providers to name, normalize and hold a space to process the roles of sociocultural contexts, socializations, and power and privilege.

For educators and supervisors of mental health professionals

Trauma and crisis education is important for counselors-in-training and other mental health professionals. Given the high prevalence of sexual violence, mental health service providers in training invariably work with clients in the journey of sexual trauma recovery. As a result, these professionals-in-training would benefit from understanding the essential components of healing from sexual trauma. It is important, therefore, that specific learning objectives on the foundational role of sociocultural contexts and socializations, power and privilege, and outcomes of disclosure be integrated into the education of mental health professionals. This will help professionals develop the skill of broaching identity and positionality factors and sociocultural contexts that impact the healing journey for survivors of sexual trauma in underrepresented groups. Moreover, educating mental health professionals about the subcategories, properties, dimensions, and processes within the cycle of trauma response would enable them to hold space for their clients to process their negative trauma reactions. Education about the cycle of trauma response also helps mental health professionals to educate their clients on potentially transferable healing strategies that could help clients gain momentum in their journey of healing from sexual trauma. In addition, integrating education on the importance of the intersection of the cycle of trauma response with the encounters with the systems and the resulting emotional burden would help counselors to become culturally responsive.

For members of the justice system

This grounded theory suggested the significant role of the survivors' sociocultural contexts and socializations, roles that determined the power and privilege associated with underrepresented identities. Because of their positionality, survivors had a continuous encounter with the system that resulted in emotional burdens. The emotional burden, or fear of inviting an encounter with the system, limited participants' ability to seek justice after an incidence of sexual violence. It is important that members of the justice system recognize the additional layer of emotional burden faced by survivors in underrepresented groups, and that they work to create a safe and non-biased space that invites survivors of sexual trauma to seek justice. It is also important for members of the justice system to recognize that internalizing blame and the tendency of taking responsibility, especially at the early stages of trauma recovery, combined with the lack of clearer understanding of consent, might impact a survivor's ability to accurately report actual events leading up to, during, and following the sexual violence encounter.

For friends, family and/or others in relationship with survivors

Disclosure was one of the important categories that emerged in the theory of healing from sexual trauma. Once disclosure of the sexual trauma encounter is made, the interpersonal outcomes of the disclosure will influence survivors' trauma response cycle and exposure to moments of relief. In this study, the social support survivors received -- from partners, family members and friends -- in naming, normalizing, and validating their sexual trauma experience was found to be valuable in the healing journey. By contrast, victim questioning and blaming following disclosure of a traumatic experience contributed to negative trauma responses. Therefore, it is important for those in close relation with survivors to provide social support through naming, accepting and normalizing the sexual violence encounter.

Future research

This grounded theory of the journey of healing from sexual trauma provided extensive data on the major factors that contribute to the trauma response cycle. As the study progressed and major categories were identified, potential areas for future studies emerged.

First, because the focus of this study was on how survivors of sexual trauma navigated their journey after the sexual trauma incident, little information was collected about the role of the pre-trauma self. The acquisition of foundational knowledge and skills to navigate and manage negative experiences before a traumatic encounter may play a role in expediting the transition to healing strategies.

Second, this study only invited participants who identified as members of an underrepresented group. The identity of the aggressor, however, and the power and privilege they held was purposefully not included as a sample selection criterion. Perhaps a shared underrepresented identity and fairly similar power and privilege status between the aggressor and the survivor would yield more and new information about the healing journey of survivors of sexual trauma. This would also be helpful to test the CBTT; a theory used as a framework for this study.

Third, only one participant in this study experienced multiple sexual violence encounters. Research on the impact of a single sexual violence encounter versus multiple encounters is needed to better understand trauma responses and helpful strategies that lead to moments of relief for survivors of repeated sexual violence encounters.

Lastly, there were hints of self-forgiveness (shifting blame from self-to-others) and forgiveness of others and the situation. Further studies on the meaning and role of forgiveness in relation to the theory described in Chapter Five would add depth to the theory.

Conclusion

Considering the higher prevalence of sexual trauma among individuals in underrepresented groups and its negative impact on the physical and mental health of survivors, it was important to develop a theory to explain the process of healing from sexual trauma for underrepresented groups. The sexual trauma survivor's journey of healing is represented as a boat floating on water, illustrating the significant components of healing. Following the sexual trauma encounter, it was important for survivors to shift their understanding of consent, which helped them name this encounter as violence. The naming, accepting and normalizing of the sexual encounter as traumatic was facilitated by survivors' exposure to new and inclusive cultures as well as the social support they received upon disclosure of their experience. The passage of time combined with intentional effort has helped survivors to focus on healing strategies.

In this grounded theory, trauma response was represented as the boat's wheel to portray its cyclical nature revolving around both positive and negative trauma responses. Social support following disclosure of sexual trauma contributed to positive trauma responses and experiences of moments of relief. The boat floats on the water, which represents the sociocultural contexts and socializations, but the water is sometimes rough and stormy, reflecting survivors' encounters with the system and the emotional burden associated with these encounters. Survivors' ability to freely explore and formulate their identities was instrumental for the development of an authentic self that contributed to their healing from sexual trauma. Survivors' experience of internal and external moments of relief kept the sail of the boat hoisted as they weathered the stormy path to recovery.

www.ingramcontent.com/pod-product-compliance
Lightning Source LLC
LaVergne TN
LVHW011929070526
838202LV00054B/4554